THE COMPLETE MACRO COOKBOOK

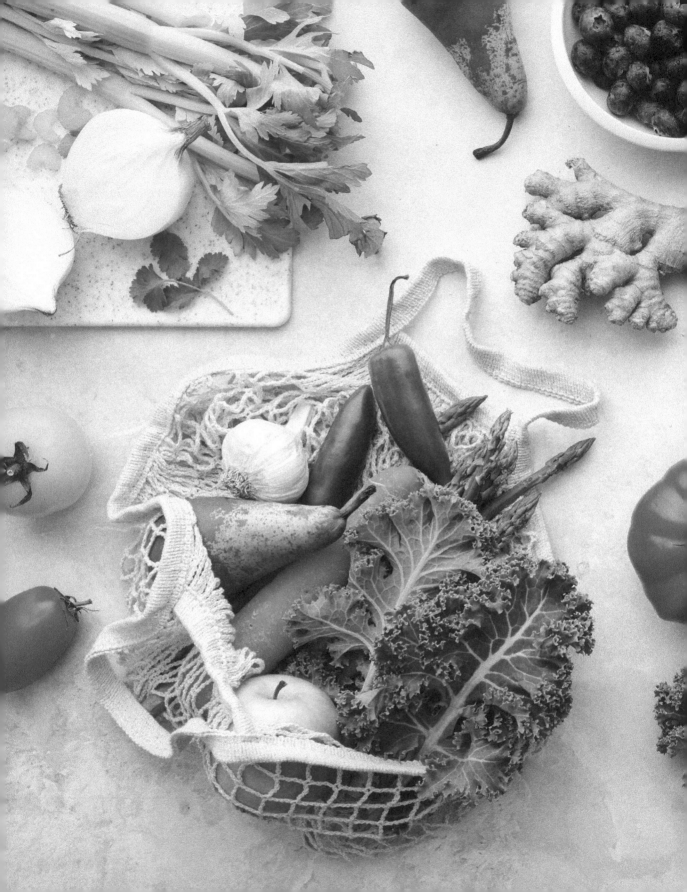

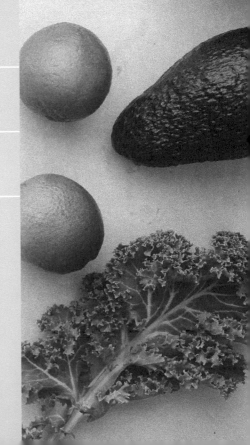

THE
COMPLETE
MACRO
COOKBOOK

WORKOUT GUIDANCE AND ROUTINES

2-WEEK MEAL PLAN FOR MUSCLE GAIN

2-WEEK MEAL PLAN FOR FAT LOSS

Brittany Scanniello, RDN

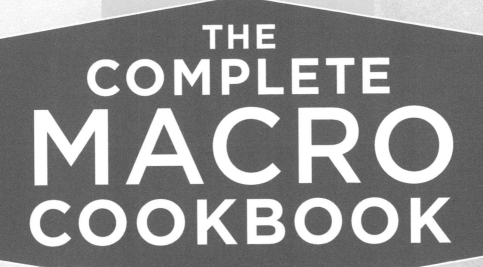

R

ROCKRIDGE
PRESS

Copyright © 2022 by Rockridge Press

First Rockridge Press trade paperback edition 2022

Rockridge Press and the Rockridge Press logo are trademarks or registered trademarks of Callisto Media Inc. and/or its affiliates in the United States and other countries and may not be used without written permission.

For general information on our other products and services, please contact our Customer Care Department within the United States at (866) 744-2665, or outside the United States at (510) 253-0500.

Some of the recipes/exercises/activities originally appeared, in different form, in *The 30-Minute Clean Eating Cookbook, Bodybuilding 30-Minute Cookbook,* and *Macro Cookbook for Beginners.*

Paperback ISBN: 978-1-63878-055-7
eBook ISBN: 978-1-63878-264-3

Manufactured in the United States of America

Interior and Cover Designer: Patricia Fabricant
Art Producer: Janice Ackerman
Editor: Marjorie DeWitt
Production Editor: Matthew Burnett
Production Manager: Martin Worthington

Photography © Darren Muir, cover left, right and bottom left and pp. ii–iii, x, 1–2, 22, 40–42, 55, 62, 85–86, 104, 110, 120, 132, 135, 159, 168; © Thomas J. Story, cover bottom right and pp. vi, 56, 81, 113, 151; © Kate Sears, pp. 47, 74, 77, 103, 107, 127, 152; © Evi Abeler, p. 78; © Laura Flippen, p. 95.

Illustration © Charlie Layton, pp. 170–172, 174–176.

Author photograph courtesy of Natalie Pigliacampo

10 9 8 7 6 5 4 3 2 1 0

This book is dedicated to those out there wanting to take control of their health, through focusing on food choice, lifestyle, and movement. I hope you find this book helpful as you begin your health journey.

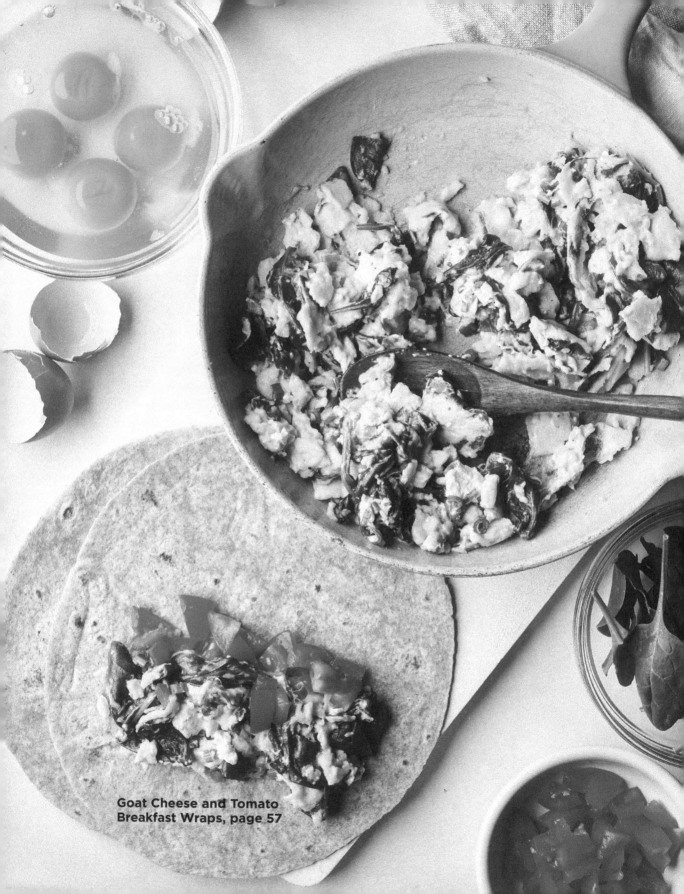

Goat Cheese and Tomato Breakfast Wraps, page 57

CONTENTS

INTRODUCTION

WHETHER WE LIKE IT OR NOT, "diet culture" is present all around us. A negative diet culture is toxic to people of all shapes and sizes, leading to disordered eating and an unhealthy relationship with food and exercise.

A newer concept making its way to the fitness and nutrition world is macronutrient counting. Macronutrient counting has taken the tech world by storm, with app after app claiming to help you lose weight by keeping track of your macros. As a registered dietitian in private and clinical practice for nearly 15 years, I have seen macronutrient counting work well for some, but I've also seen it used in an unhealthy manner. Improving my clients' relationships with food is something I work on daily and is one of the many reasons I got into nutrition in the first place, and is why I chose to write this book.

The macro way of eating emphasizes food choice, balance, and complete meals. It allows for flexibility, encourages a focus on whole foods from all food groups, and is a way of eating that can last a lifetime. The term "macro" can mean big picture, and this way of eating is exactly that. A macronutrient-counting diet looks at your daily intake and how all the individual foods you consume work together to meet your daily nutrition goals. I have seen this lifestyle work firsthand, improving people's relationship with food while also helping them meet health goals like fat loss or muscle gain in an effective, efficient way.

In this book, I have outlined everything you need to transition to a healthy macro-counting lifestyle. You'll learn what exactly macronutrient counting is and why it works. I'll go into detail on how counting your macronutrients compares to other diets (new and old), as well as who it may be a good fit for and who may require additional help from a registered dietitian or healthcare provider to guarantee success. I have included two 14-day meal and exercise plans tailored to specific health goals with additional recipes to keep you going along the way.

This book is here to help those who are stuck in a health rut or who are looking for something they can maintain for a lifetime. I want to encourage a healthy relationship with food and show you how to incorporate a variety of foods and food groups into a wholesome, balanced meal plan while still meeting your health and fitness goals. Having this book as a resource will prepare you for bettering your food choices, creating complete meals, and implementing an exercise routine that is doable, not daunting. I look forward to sharing this journey with you.

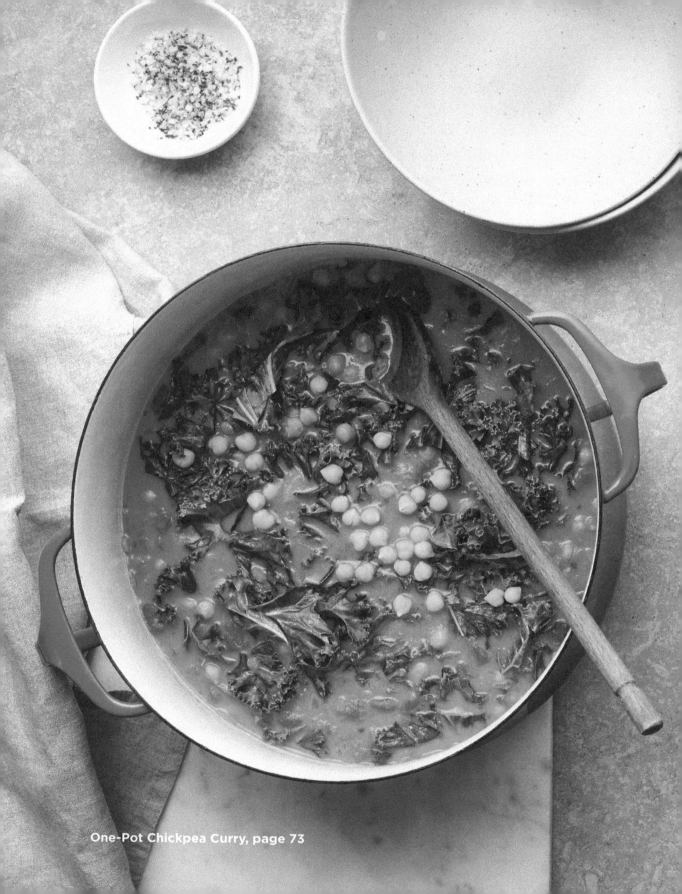

One-Pot Chickpea Curry, page 73

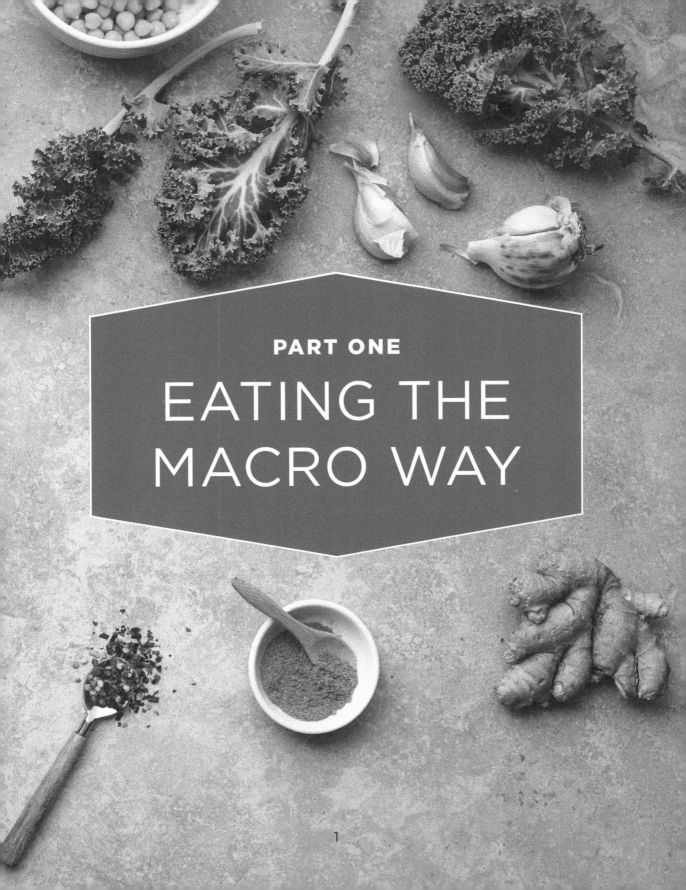

PART ONE
EATING THE MACRO WAY

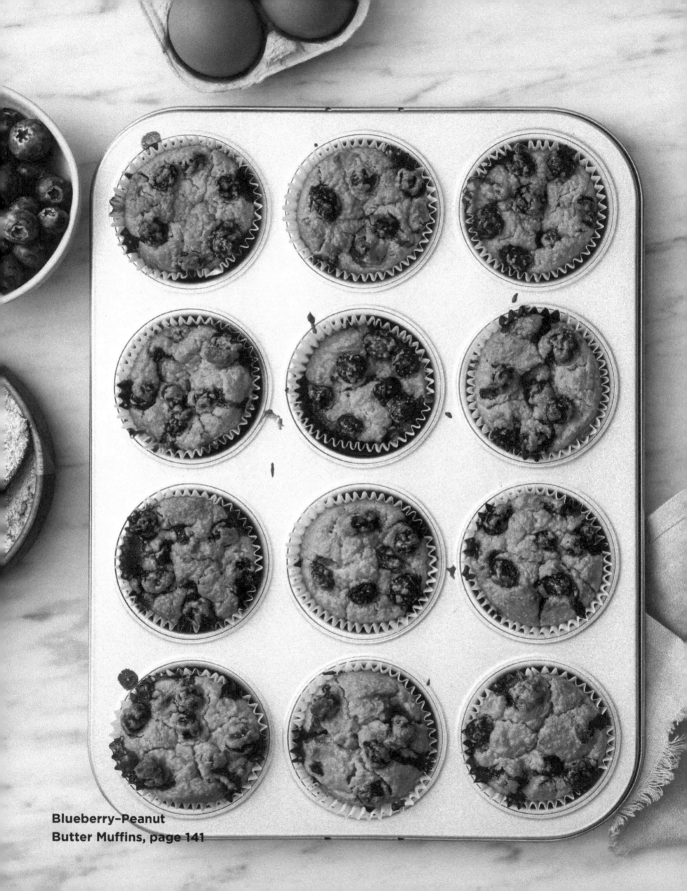

**Blueberry-Peanut
Butter Muffins, page 141**

ALL ABOUT THE MACRO DIET

Taking control of your health is something we all strive for, but often it's much easier said than done. It takes time and dedication. I'm here to provide you with the basic knowledge to kick-start a new way of thinking about food. We will cover the macro way of eating, which is a lifestyle, not a diet.

Have Your Cake—and Eat It, Too

You may have heard of macro counting at your local gym, seen it on a magazine cover, or talked about it with a friend who's always up on the latest nutrition trends. Maybe you haven't heard of macro counting, but you're here because you're looking for a lifelong solution to improve your health and other diets haven't worked for you—they were too restrictive, left you feeling unsatisfied, or just weren't sustainable long-term. Whatever the reason, welcome!

Macronutrient counting can help anyone who is looking to make more informed food choices and better understand how foods impact their individual health goals. Whether you're aiming to lose weight, gain muscle, or focus on weight maintenance, the macro diet—also referred to as "flexible dieting"—helps you make choices that are completely customized to your goals.

The macro diet is not a one-size-fits-all approach to dieting. In fact, it's less of a diet and more of a lifestyle, a way of eating that's meant to satisfy, not deprive. It's not intended to eliminate total food groups, as other diets may advise or require. The goal is to focus on whole foods, to understand how they fit into your nutrition and fitness goals, and to know where your calories and macronutrients come from and the effect each one has on your body.

WHAT IS THE MACRO DIET?

Some in the health and fitness world might say that counting macros is quickly becoming the new counting calories—but what does that actually mean?

The macro diet takes calorie counting one step further. For this diet, you count the macronutrients (macros)—carbohydrates, protein, and fat, measured in grams—that you're eating in each meal and snack throughout the day. To break it down a bit further, you find your target macro ratios (for example, 50 percent of your total calories from carbohydrates, 25 percent from protein, and 25 percent from fat) and plan your food choices to meet those macro intake goals.

DIET FLEXIBILITY. Unlike other popular diets, macro tracking does not force you to cut out entire food groups or specific foods. If the foods you choose fit into your daily macro goals, indulge and enjoy!

IMPROVED UNDERSTANDING OF THE FOODS YOU EAT. Tracking your dietary intake for any length of time can provide you with a lot of information. Sometimes this information can be eye-opening. Some foods may fuel your workouts better than others, while some may keep you satisfied longer. Meanwhile, other foods may cause undesirable outcomes such as bloating or gas. Information is power. The more you know, the easier it is to make tailored adjustments to reach your health goals.

WELL-ROUNDED DIET. The main principle of the macro diet is to eat whole foods from all food groups. This equates to a well-rounded diet and ensures a variety of vitamins and minerals.

TARGETED MUSCLE GAIN. If you're looking to build lean muscle while maintaining a healthy weight, it's imperative to eat enough protein. Adequate protein is required to build muscle, to repair muscle, and to support existing muscle.

FAT LOSS. Each macronutrient has a different effect on your metabolism. When consuming specific ratios of macronutrients, you can indirectly control your appetite, support lean body mass, and maintain energy levels, all while losing body fat.

WHY DOES IT WORK?

Everyone starting the macro diet will begin with a target macro ratio. Various online calculators can determine this—or even better, you can consult with a dietitian who can help get you started with the most appropriate macro ratio based on your body type, your fitness and nutrition goals, your activity level, and your medical history. When used correctly, a macro diet keeps you feeling fuller longer, balances your energy levels, and keeps your cravings at bay. The macro diet is completely customizable for your goals and body type, allowing you to adjust accordingly if you're not seeing the results you want.

WHO IS IT FOR?

While the macro diet does offer flexibility, it doesn't come without work. If you're someone who thrives on structure and likes to change up what you eat, then look no further! Healthy individuals who want to lose fat, gain muscle mass, or focus on weight maintenance while enjoying a wide variety of foods have come to the right place. Individuals with underlying health concerns, such as diabetes or a history of disordered eating, should consult with their healthcare provider to make sure the macro diet is a good fit. This is not to say that those with health concerns are unable to follow a macro way of eating; these individuals will just require additional support to ensure they are fully meeting their nutrition needs.

The Building Blocks of Body Composition

Counting macros can help you reach various health goals. The idea is to base your diet on whole foods, learn how they fit your macro targets, and understand what effect each macronutrient and food has on your body.

CALORIES

What is a calorie? While the question may sound simple, the answer can be a bit complicated. A calorie is a way to measure energy. In the context of nutrition, a calorie is the energy you take in from foods or beverages you consume. It also refers to the energy you expend during physical activity.

Having the right quantity of calories is key for survival and good health. What can make calories tricky is the fact that each person requires a different number of them to meet their daily requirements. An individual's energy needs can be dependent on their age, gender, weight, height, body shape, physical activity, and muscle mass, to name just a few key factors. When your calorie consumption is unbalanced—whether it be too low or too high—health problems can arise.

When it comes to weight gain and weight loss, the simple adage of "calories in versus calories out" has some truth behind it, but it's not that easy. While total calories consumed matters when it comes to our health goals, it's also important to focus on the types of foods supplying those calories.

MACRONUTRIENTS

Macronutrients (macros) are the three primary nutrient groups that provide the energy our bodies need to perform activities and sustain life. These groups consist of carbohydrates, protein, and fat. Each macronutrient plays a distinct role in nutrition and has a unique impact on our bodies. Adequate protein intake is critical for building muscle, repairing muscle after workouts, and supporting existing muscle. Carbohydrates provide us with the energy we need, whether for immediate use or stored in our muscles and liver for later. Fats are vital not only for energy, but for hormone production, proper nutrient absorption, and maintaining body temperature.

It's important to note that everyone requires different amounts of each macronutrient to perform their daily functions. Understanding how your body responds to each macronutrient allows you to customize a diet plan that provides your body with exactly what it needs to thrive.

DIET QUALITY

Diet quality refers to a diversified and balanced diet, which provides energy and all essential nutrients to sustain a healthy, active lifestyle. Unlike other eating plans, the macro diet does not restrict any foods or food groups. Rather, macro counting is based on the concept that not all calories are created equal. When working to meet health goals like fat loss, muscle gain, or weight maintenance, focusing on the types of calories eaten is more important than the total number of calories consumed.

If counting only calories, you may mindlessly reach for a 200-calorie snack pack from your local vending machine. When counting macros, you'll rethink how you're eating, opting for a less processed, whole food choice to better meet your daily macro goals (such as an apple and handful of almonds instead to meet your carb and protein goals, respectively).

That being said, if you really want that bowl of ice cream or slice of grandma's apple pie—do it! Counting macros doesn't mean you have to deprive yourself when it comes to food choices. What it does mean is that you should aim for whole ingredients and real foods most of the time. For the remainder, say 20 percent of the time, enjoy your favorite treat. This 80/20 Rule is one I live by, and it is something that we will be going over in detail later in this chapter.

A Closer Look at Macronutrients

As we've discussed, the three macronutrients to keep track of are protein, carbohydrates, and fat. Once you determine the most appropriate daily macro goals for you, the next step is to ensure that you're choosing the best foods to meet those targets.

PROTEIN

Protein is vital. Without it, our bodies won't have the building blocks they need to function properly. Proteins are critical for building and repairing muscle, as well as creating essential hormones and enzymes throughout our body.

Each gram of protein is equivalent to 4 calories. A few protein-rich foods include:

- **LEAN MEAT:** 4 ounces of grilled skinless chicken breast provides 35 grams of protein.

- **SALMON:** 4 ounces of grilled salmon provides 30 grams of protein.

- **EGG:** 1 egg provides 7 grams of protein.

- **GREEK YOGURT:** a 6-ounce serving of Greek yogurt contains 17 grams of protein.

- **LENTILS:** 1 cup of cooked lentils provided 18 grams of protein.

- **PEANUT BUTTER:** 2 tablespoons of peanut butter provides 8 grams of protein.

When it comes to protein supplements, these can come from a variety of sources, including eggs, dairy (whey or casein), and plants (soy, pea, or hemp). While a protein supplement is not necessary, some people find them helpful to meet their daily protein intake goals. Like other supplements, protein powders aren't regulated by the U.S. Food and Drug Administration (FDA) for safety and contaminants. It's important to read food labels, know where your product is coming from, and watch out for added sugars, fillers, and artificial flavorings.

CARBOHYDRATES

Carbohydrates provide glucose, the preferred energy source for your brain, central nervous system, and muscles.

Carbs are further classified into two types: simple or complex. Simple carbs are digested or broken down by the body much faster, resulting in a brief spike in energy, often referred to as a "sugar rush." This type of carb, typically added to foods in the form of sugar or corn syrup, is often considered unhealthy.

Fruit and dairy also contain simple carbs, but both can be consumed in a healthy manner, as fruit contains fiber, and dairy contains fat and protein alongside carbohydrates. When you have a combination of nutrients together, the simple carb is less likely to produce such a rapid rise in blood sugar.

Complex carbs are generally found in whole grains such as whole-wheat bread, brown rice, oatmeal, quinoa, and beans. Complex carbs take longer for the body to break down, resulting in consistent blood sugar levels and lasting energy.

Like protein, each gram of carbohydrate is equal to 4 calories. Some quality carbohydrates include:

- **QUINOA:** 1 cup of cooked quinoa provides 40 grams of carbs.

- **BLACK BEANS:** 1 cup of cooked black beans provides 44 grams of carbs.

- **BERRIES:** 1 cup of berries provides about 20 grams of carbs.

- **OATMEAL:** 1 cup of cooked oatmeal provides 28 grams of carbs.

- **BANANA:** 1 medium banana provides 28 grams of carbs.

FAT

Historically a villain in the "diet" world, fat gained a bad rap due to being the most calorically dense of the macronutrients at 9 calories per gram. But fats are not the enemy. In fact, they are crucial for meeting your daily needs of fat-soluble vitamins (A, D, E, and K), hormone regulation, and temperature control.

Like carbs, fats fall into different categories. One category is saturated fats, often referred to as "bad fats." Saturated fats tend to raise low-density lipoprotein (LDL) cholesterol, increasing your risk of heart disease and stroke. A saturated fat is one that is solid at room temperature: Think red meat, cheese, and butter.

Trans fats are another type of saturated fat. These have also been found to contribute to an increased risk of stroke, heart disease, and type 2 diabetes. A common trans fat frequently found in store-bought baked goods, shortening, and fried foods is labeled as "partially hydrogenated oil." Trans fats should be avoided as much as possible.

Unsaturated fats, also known as "heart-healthy" or "good" fats are the ones to aim for. Unsaturated fats can reduce inflammation and lower LDL cholesterol, among other benefits.

Some key unsaturated fats to focus on include:

- **AVOCADO:** ½ medium avocado provides 12 grams of fat.

- **FLAXSEED:** 1 tablespoon of flaxseed provides 2 grams of fat.

- **WALNUTS:** 1 ounce of walnuts (about 14 halves) provides 18 grams of fat.

- **OLIVE OIL:** 1 tablespoon of olive oil provides 14 grams of fat.

- **SALMON:** a 3-ounce serving of salmon provides 6 grams of fat.

MICRONUTRIENTS

Micronutrients, or vitamins and minerals, are vital to good health, disease prevention, and overall well-being. Most micronutrients are not produced by the body and therefore must be provided by your diet. While everyone needs an array of micronutrients for good health, here are some important ones to focus on.

IRON is critical for cognitive development and oxygen delivery throughout your body. High-iron foods include lean meat, seafood, poultry, beans, nuts, and iron-fortified cereals.

VITAMIN D is needed for bone strengthening, immune support, muscle, and nerve function. Very few foods contain vitamin D naturally, so fortified foods are your best option. Look for fortified milks and eggs.

VITAMIN A supports vision and proper immune function. Foods with high amounts of vitamin A include salmon, organ meats, leafy greens, and orange and yellow vegetables.

CALCIUM works with vitamin D to maintain strong bones. You can find calcium in dairy products and certain vegetables like kale, broccoli, and spinach.

ZINC is necessary to keep your immune system strong and healthy. It's prevalent in many foods, including poultry, red meat, oysters, beans, nuts, whole grains, and dairy.

Bottom line, variety is key. Eating varied sources of protein, fat, whole grains, fruits, and vegetables will give your body the macro- and micronutrients it needs to do what you need it to.

BEVERAGES

Water remains one of the most important nutrients. Whether you're training or not, in good health or working to get there, maintaining your hydration is essential. Water keeps our muscles and joints fluid, helps detoxify our bodies, and aids in muscle repair, healing, and growth.

Convenient as it would be, there is not an exact amount of water each of us needs daily. Therefore, you should always monitor the color of your urine. When it's clear, you're likely well hydrated. If your urine is dark, thick, slow flowing, or bright green, these are all signs of dehydration. If you're a numbers person, you can use this quick calculation to determine a daily goal: 45 milliliters (mL) x your bodyweight in kilograms = total mL of water to consume daily. If you're participating in weight or endurance training, this volume increases. You should speak with your healthcare provider or trainer to ensure you're hydrating adequately.

Most fluids contribute toward your daily fluid intake and rehydration, but with differing levels of effectiveness. The exception here is alcohol and beverages with large amounts of caffeine, as both have a diuretic effect on the body. For most individuals, any combination of beverages (excluding alcohol and caffeine- and sugar-filled options) throughout the day should be sufficient for meeting your hydration needs.

THE 80/20 LIFESTYLE

The idea here is to make sure that 80 percent of your total intake is coming from clean, nutrient-dense foods. The remaining 20 percent can be more flexible, to allow you to plan around dinner parties or celebrations, travel days, or days when just don't feel like counting your macros. This gives you a chance to have an "off day" and some freedom, as life happens and sometimes our plans don't work out.

In broader terms, the 80/20 lifestyle holds you accountable for sticking to your eating plan of wholesome, nutritious foods 80 percent of the time. For the remaining 20 percent, allow yourself to indulge and don't feel guilty about it. This is roughly 4 meals a week (if following a 3 meals/day routine) where you can let loose a bit and eat what feels good. Macro counting is about a sustainable, lifelong way of eating. Too many people face difficulty with diet plans because they're too restrictive and boring. The macro lifestyle is about variety and making it work for you.

How to Calculate Your Macros

Rather than struggling to determine your ideal calorie goal, macro split, and macro targets, I always suggest working with a registered dietitian or qualified healthcare provider to determine what's right for you.

If that isn't feasible, you can always use an online macro calculator as a starting point. To do this, you'll be asked for biometrics such as your age, gender, height, weight, and health goals. The calculator will then use this information to determine your ideal macro split. A favorite of mine is the IIFYM calculator (https://www.iifym.com/macro-calculator/). I want to stress this again: Everybody is unique and will respond differently to different macro splits. Keep a journal to track your progress and note what is working for you as you begin your journey.

Now, if doing it the old-fashioned way by putting pen to paper, follow these steps:

1. DETERMINE YOUR BASAL METABOLIC RATE (BMR)

Everyone's BMR is the minimum number of calories you must consume daily to sustain life. Your BMR is different from your neighbor's or your friend's and is influenced by your weight, total body composition, and sex. To determine your precise BMR, I suggest getting a basal metabolic rate test at your local gym. If that isn't possible, you can use the following calculation for a rough estimate:

Women: (4.536 x weight in pounds) + (15.88 x height in inches) – (5 x age) – 161 = BMR

Men: (4.536 x weight in pounds) + (15.88 x height in inches) – (5 x age) + 5 = BMR

2. FIGURE OUT YOUR ACTIVITY LEVEL

Once you have determined your BMR, take this number and multiply it by your physical activity level (PAL). Typical PAL ranges from 1.2 (sedentary) to 1.9 (extremely active). Here's how to calculate your caloric needs depending on your physical activity level:

- Sedentary (little to no exercise) = BMR x 1.2

- Lightly active (light exercise one to three days per week) = BMR x 1.375

- Moderately active (moderate exercise six to seven days a week) = BMR x 1.55

- Very active (hard exercise every day or exercising twice per day) = BMR x 1.725

- Extra active (hard exercise two or more times per day, training for a marathon or triathlon, or any activity where endurance is critical) = BMR x 1.9

3. CHOOSE YOUR MACRO SPLIT

Once you've established your daily caloric needs, what's next? Choosing your macro split determines where your calories are coming from between carbs, fat, and protein. The ratio in which you split your daily macros can promote muscle gain, fat loss, or weight maintenance.

The goal with muscle gain is to ensure that you're consuming sufficient carbs to fuel your workouts, enough protein to build and repair your muscles, and just enough fat to maintain healthy hormone levels. When muscle gain is your goal, I recommend splitting your macros as follows:

- 40 to 50 percent carbs

- 25 to 35 percent protein

- 20 to 25 percent fat

For fat loss, you want to focus on specific macro ratios while maintaining a slight calorie deficit from your BMR. A good rule of thumb is to consume 10 to 15 percent fewer calories than what you burn every day. Here are my recommended ratios for fat loss:

- 20 to 30 percent carbs (If you're very active or extra active according to PAL, you will need a higher amount of carbs.)

- 30 to 40 percent protein

- 30 to 40 percent fat

Upping your protein macro goal to 40% or higher can provide extra satiety and works well for some while trying to lose weight, but individual tolerance varies. Adjust your protein intake gradually, especially at these higher levels, and contact your healthcare provider if you experience any negative side effects.

When weight maintenance is your goal, I recommend splitting your macros as outlined:

- 35 to 45 percent carbs

- 25 to 35 percent protein

- 25 to 35 percent fat

4. CALCULATE THE GRAMS FOR EACH MACRO

As your final step in determining your macros, calculate how many grams of each macronutrient you need by multiplying your total daily calories by your protein, carbs, and fat percentages as outlined by which health goal you are looking to achieve. Once you've determined these numbers, you then divide the protein and carbs number by 4 and the fat number by 9. You can find examples of this on page 20.

How to Meal Plan around Macros

When getting started with macro counting, it can feel overwhelming. Whether you're preparing meals for just yourself or for a larger household, it takes time, preparation, and a plan. My advice here is to persevere! You will thank yourself later. It just requires a little time, and you will soon settle into a new routine and never look back.

If you know that meal planning is not for you, don't close the book now. You too can count macros; it may just look a little different. I'd recommend choosing some easy go-tos to always have on hand on those days where any sort of planning goes out the window, so you still have something to fall back on. For example, frozen chicken breasts or fish fillets; fresh fruit and veggies; and whole grains such as brown rice, quinoa, or beans. A simple dinner can come together quickly with some grilled chicken breast, steamed broccoli, and a side of quinoa.

If you need something different every day, that's okay, too! Meal planning and prepping may be more up your alley. If this is the case, I recommend setting aside time every Sunday to meal plan, grocery shop, and prep what you can, so you're ready to go once the week starts.

PORTION CONTROL

A food scale will allow you to more accurately assess the portions you're consuming. However, a food scale is not mandatory for macro counting. There are some simple tricks to help you estimate your serving sizes.

- Three ounces of cooked meat, fish, or poultry is roughly the size of a deck of cards.

- One cup of cooked pasta or whole grains should be equivalent to the size of your closed fist.

- One teaspoon of oil is about the size of your thumb.

- A medium-size fruit is the size of a tennis ball.

- One cup of veggies is close to the size of a baseball.

- For nut butters, a ping pong ball is equivalent to 2 tablespoons.

- One ounce of cheese is the size of a pair of dice.

THE ROLE OF FITNESS

Do you have to exercise to lose weight? The answer is no. However, exercise brings with it a whole host of health benefits, along with confidence, endorphins, and general improvement to your day-to-day life.

In the meal plans in chapter 2, you'll find specific exercises and routines paired with each day, which can boost the benefits of the macro diet.

FAT LOSS

If fat loss is your primary health goal, high-intensity interval training (HIIT) a few times a week is at the top of my list of recommended exercises. HIIT promotes fat loss by offering a solid workout in a short period of time while keeping your post-exercise burn at an all-time high. You continue to burn calories even for a short period after the workout is complete.

An example of a quick form of HIIT training is a Tabata routine. Tabata focuses on eight 20-second rounds of exercise at an all-out intensity with 10 seconds of rest between rounds. Pick an exercise that will get your heart rate up quickly (e.g., squat jumps, burpees, jump rope, sprints).

MUSCLE GAIN

Bottom line: Resistance training builds muscle. A 2019 review in the *International Journal of Environmental Research and Public Health* found that doing multiple sets of resistance exercises while elevating your heart rate was the best combo to promote muscle gain.

An example workout may include 3 to 6 different sets, each 6 to 12 reps, with 1 minute of rest in between. Exercises that focus on muscle gain include lunges, squats, shoulder presses, and push-ups.

FOOD TIMING

Macro counting does not come without hard work. It takes time to plan your meals, prep food ahead of time, and log the foods you're consuming. Choosing what to eat is about balance, rather than timing. I want you to be successful, and I want you to eat the foods you choose when you want to eat them.

If you're looking to plan meals that work for your daily routine, consider pairing carbs and protein after training to aid in recovery and a mix of protein, fats, and fiber for dinner to promote fullness.

PLATEAUS

Plateaus happen to all of us and for different reasons. They could be related to inaccurate tracking, metabolic adaptation, dehydration, suboptimal fiber intake, or exercise routine fatigue, to name a few. Therefore, I cannot stress enough how important it is to track your progress and note what is and is not working for you.

If you have hit a plateau, there are ways to work through it. I'll go over some troubleshooting tips later in this chapter that you can address with a registered dietitian or healthcare provider to help you start making progress again.

REST AND INJURY PREVENTION

Overtraining is real, and it can have serious side effects. If we don't allow our bodies to fully recover between workouts, our bodies begin to break. Ensuring adequate sleep, stress management, and nutrition is critical to staying safe and healthy. Listen to your body and be honest with yourself before every workout.

MEAL PREPPING

Meal prepping is not something you have to do, but it does make tracking macros a bit easier. By starting each week prepared, you're setting yourself up for success. I often recommend doing as much of your meal prep on Sundays as possible, so it is easy to grab and go during the rest of the week, but this is not imperative. Just do what works best for you.

Troubleshooting

We talked about it earlier. Plateaus happen and are frustrating. If you're experiencing a plateau and not seeing the results you desire, it could be due to a variety of reasons:

INCORRECT MACRO RATIOS. This is extremely important to get right, as it is tailored to you. If you're not seeing the results you want, schedule an appointment with a registered dietitian or your healthcare provider to discuss your health goals and have them help you find the best macro ratios for you.

INACCURATE MACRO TRACKING. Sometimes we may be eating more than we think. Every bite, taste, and nibble counts, so it's important to track everything. If you're not tracking everything, you may be consuming more than your macro goals are set for.

METABOLIC ADAPTATION. Our bodies are intelligent. If you've been following a similar macro split and exercise routine for a while, it may be time to mix it up. Sometimes just a quick increase or decrease in total calories and/or a shift in macro ratios will be what your body needs to start making progress again.

INSUFFICIENT WATER INTAKE. Water promotes proper digestion. The more we drink, the better our body works through the food we consume. If we don't drink enough water, our digestive system tends to slow and works much less efficiently.

STRESS. Stress causes a spike in the hormone cortisol, which has a negative effect on our total calorie burn. When our stress is properly managed and under control, our body regulates its cortisol levels and burns calories much more effectively.

EXERCISE FATIGUE. Mix it up! If you feel you're running yourself to death on the treadmill, pick up some weights instead. Be sure to implement a variety of different types of exercise on a weekly basis. Think HIIT, cardio, resistance training, yoga, and Pilates—all of which have outstanding benefits to our bodies and health in their own way.

Tracking your macros simply means logging the foods you eat on a website, in an app, or in a food journal. Some of my favorite apps include MacroFactor, Lose It!, MyFitnessPal, and My Macros+, which are all very user-friendly and do a lot of the tracking for you. You just input the food item and serving size, and your total macros are logged and accounted for. However, a regular food journal is fine, too.

The art of tracking is to hold yourself accountable and know exactly where you are at any given point of the day. There will be days when you don't hit your exact macro target for each of the macronutrients. That's okay! What's important is that you're staying in the general range, as your target macros are there specifically for you to meet the health goals you have set forth at the beginning of your journey.

About the Meal Plans

In chapter 2, I'll outline some 14-day meal plans, shopping guides, and meal prep tips and tricks. All will be geared toward specific goals, whether that be fat loss or muscle gain.

FAT LOSS

As we discussed earlier, if your goal is to lose fat, I recommend splitting your macros as follows.

- 20 to 30 percent carbs

- 30 to 40 percent protein

- 30 to 40 percent fat

When aiming for fat loss, it's important to focus on specific macro ratios, while at the same time ensuring these are based on a calorie amount 10 to 15 percent less than what you determined your BMR + PAL was earlier in this chapter.

For example, if you determined your daily calorie requirement (BMR + PAL) was 1,900 calories, then your new daily calorie allotment to promote fat loss would be 1,710 (10 percent deficit). Your macro breakdown would look like this:

- **CARB (25 PERCENT OF CALORIES/4 CALORIES PER GRAM):** 107 grams/day

- **PROTEIN (40 PERCENT OF CALORIES/4 CALORIES PER GRAM):** 171 grams/day

- **FAT (35 PERCENT OF CALORIES/9 CALORIES PER GRAM):** 67 grams/day

For your activity, use a variety of exercises to prevent injury and burnout. Also be sure to incorporate rest days to ensure your body has time to recover. If aiming for fat loss and your activity level is very active (five or more days a week), you'll need to bump up your total carb intake, while maintaining total protein, resulting in a slight decrease in total fat to maintain your macro splits accordingly.

MUSCLE GAIN

If looking to gain muscle but not necessarily drop weight, I recommend splitting your macros as follows:

- 40 to 50 percent carbs

- 25 to 35 percent protein

- 20 to 25 percent fat

To promote muscle gain, you must consume enough carbs to fuel your workouts, adequate protein to allow your muscles to build and repair, and just enough fat to maintain healthy hormone levels. Implement resistance training in addition to stretching and adequate rest.

As an example, if your daily calorie requirement is 2,200 calories, your macro breakdown would look like this:

- **CARB (45 PERCENT OF CALORIES/4 CALORIES PER GRAM):** 248 grams/day

- **PROTEIN (35 PERCENT OF CALORIES/4 CALORIES PER GRAM):** 193 grams/day

- **FAT (20 PERCENT OF CALORIES/9 CALORIES PER GRAM):** 49 grams/day

FAT LOSS VS. MUSCLE GAIN RECIPES

Throughout the rest of this book, you'll see a variety of recipes. Each recipe is labeled for fat loss or muscle gain. The recipes can be used interchangeably for either health goal, so don't count one out just because it says "Muscle Gain" if your goal happens to be fat loss. I provide tips with each recipe on ways to make it fit for you. The tips may be methods to increase protein via a protein powder or other high-protein add-ins; they may offer options for cutting out some fat calories; or I may have you add fiber to help with satiety and digestion. Whatever your goal, we have you covered with recipes for breakfast, lunch, dinner, snacks, dessert, and even DIY pantry staples that you can feel good about.

Maintaining Your Results

You did it—congratulations! You met your health goal. But now what? This is what is so great about the macro diet. You can and should maintain this way of eating, as it can be lifelong. The only thing to adjust is your macro split, since maintaining your results is a new phase.

If your goal is to maintain your current weight, I recommend splitting your macros as follows:

- 35 to 45 percent carbs

- 25 to 35 percent protein

- 25 to 35 percent fat

  An example of a 2,000-calorie diet would look like this:

- **CARB (40 PERCENT OF CALORIES/4 CALORIES PER GRAM):**
  200 grams/day

- **PROTEIN (30 PERCENT OF CALORIES/4 CALORIES PER GRAM):**
  150 grams/day

- **FAT (30 PERCENT OF CALORIES/9 CALORIES PER GRAM):** 67 grams/day

  If you "fall off the wagon," get back on. If you've gained a few pounds and want to trim down, go back to the beginning of the chapter, determine your BMR + PAL, and recalculate your new macro split according to your new goal!

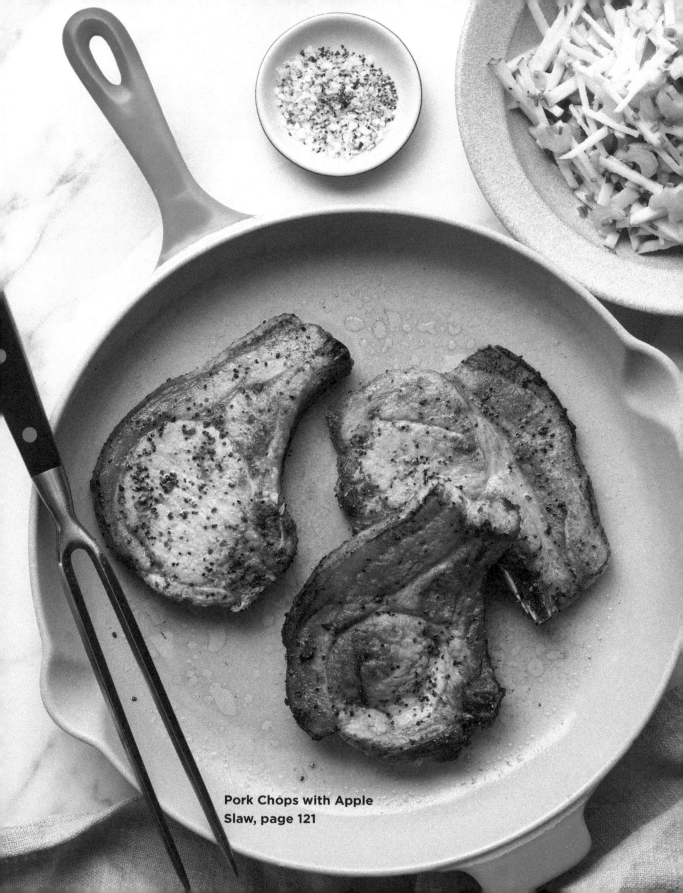

**Pork Chops with Apple
Slaw, page 121**

2

MEAL PLANS FOR FAT LOSS AND MUSCLE GAIN

Meal planning and meal prep can make tracking your macros a bit easier, especially when you're first getting started. The same goes for exercise. When you begin each week with a plan of what foods you'll eat and what exercises you'll perform, you're setting yourself up for success. I have outlined some of my favorite meal and exercise plans to help you begin your journey. At the end of the week, "Reader's Choice" offers opportunities to finish any leftovers you've accumulated or vary your routine with different foods.

I have created a meal plan for 1,600 calories to promote fat loss with a macronutrient breakdown of 30% calories from carbohydrate, 35% of calories from protein, and 35% of calories from fat.

To cover those of you with a goal of muscle gain, I have based that meal plan on a 2000-calorie intake with a macro breakdown consisting of 45% of calories from carbohydrate, 30% of calories from protein, and 25% of calorie from fat.

As mentioned throughout this book, you can use these meal plans as guides when planning your meals and snacks. Be sure to adjust accordingly if your specific calorie and macro goals fall at slightly different numbers.

14-Day Plan for Fat Loss: Week 1

	BREAKFAST	SNACK	LUNCH	SNACK	DINNER	WORKOUT
MONDAY	Eat-Your-Greens Smoothie (page 45) + 2 scoops protein powder	2 Perfect Hard-Boiled Eggs (page 156)	Chickpea and Pear Kale Salad (page 84). Can add 4 ounces grilled chicken, fish, or tofu for additional protein.	5-Minute Guac (page 164) + raw veggies of your choice	Salmon Poke Bowls (page 97)	Fat Loss Strength Training Routine 1 (page 170)
TUESDAY	Eat-Your-Greens Smoothie (leftover)	Carrots + 2 table-spoons Rainbow Hummus (page 160)	Crunchy Kale and Salmon Salad (page 98) *(using leftover salmon from dinner)*	Celery sticks + 2 table-spoons Creamy Peanut Butter (page 157)	Macro-Friendly Lamb Tagine (page 129) + a low-carb side such as ¾ cup steamed veggies or side salad	Cardio
WEDNESDAY	Fancy Avocado Toast (page 53) + 2 eggs	Celery sticks + 2 table-spoons Creamy Peanut Butter (leftover)	Macro-Friendly Lamb Tagine (leftover)	2 Perfect Hard-Boiled Eggs (leftover)	30-Minute Veggie Risotto (page 64)	HIIT

	BREAKFAST	SNACK	LUNCH	SNACK	DINNER	WORKOUT
THURSDAY	Chia-Matcha Smoothie Bowls (page 46) + 2 scoops protein powder	Carrots + 2 table-spoons Rainbow Hummus	30-Minute Veggie Risotto (leftover)	5-Minute Guac (leftover) + veggie sticks	Weeknight Steak Salad (page 117)	Rest + Recover Day
FRIDAY	PB&B Overnight Oats (page 51)	2 Perfect Hard-Boiled Eggs (leftover) or Chia-Matcha Smoothie Bowls (leftover)	Weeknight Steak Salad (leftover)	5-Minute Guac (leftover) + veggie sticks	Blackened Fish Tacos (page 91)	Fat Loss Strength Training Routine 2 (page 171)
SATURDAY	Summer Veggie Frittata (page 59) + whole-wheat tortilla	Apple + 2 table-spoons Creamy Peanut Butter (leftover)	**READER'S CHOICE**	PB&B Overnight Oats (leftover)	**READER'S CHOICE**	Cardio
SUNDAY	**READER'S CHOICE**	Carrots + 2 table-spoons Rainbow Hummus (leftover)	**READER'S CHOICE**	5-Minute Guac (leftover) + veggies sticks	Turkey-Stuffed Peppers (page 99)	Rest + Recover Day

SHOPPING LIST

PRODUCE

- Apple, green (1)
- Apple, color of choice (1)
- Asparagus (4 spears)
- Avocados (6)
- Banana (1)
- Bell peppers (3)
- Berries (¼ cup)
- Broccolini (½ bunch)
- Cabbage, red (¼ head)
- Carrots (12)
- Celery (3 stalks)
- Cherry tomatoes (1 cup)
- Cilantro, fresh (1 bunch)
- Cucumber (½)
- Garlic (6 cloves)

- Jalapeño
  (1; optional)
- Kale (2 cups)
- Lemons (2)
- Limes (2)

- Mushrooms (½ cup)
- Onion (1)
- Pear (1)
- Shallot (1)

- Spinach (3 cups)
- Tomato (1)
- Zucchini (½)

DAIRY AND EGGS

- Eggs, large (9)
- Goat cheese, crumbled (¼ cup)
- Greek yogurt (2 ounces)

- Heavy (whipping) cream (2 ounces)
- Milk or unsweetened nondairy alternative (30 ounces)

- Parmesan cheese (½ cup)

MEAT AND SEAFOOD

- Bacon (2 slices)
- Flank steak (12 ounces)

- Lamb, ground (8 ounces)
- Mahi-mahi or halibut (12 ounces)

- Smoked salmon (8 ounces)
- Turkey, ground (8 ounces)

FROZEN

- Blueberries (½ cup; can buy fresh instead)
- Edamame (½ cup)

- Peach slices (½ cup; can buy fresh instead)

- Pineapple (½ cup; can buy fresh instead)

HERBS AND SPICES

- Black pepper
- Cayenne pepper
- Cinnamon, ground

- Cumin, ground
- Garam masala
- Garlic powder

- Paprika
- Red pepper flakes
- Salt

PANTRY

- Arborio rice
  (½ cup)

- Broth, unsalted
  vegetable
  or chicken

- Chia seeds

- Chickpeas
  (2 [15-ounce] cans)

- Diced tomatoes
  (1 [15-ounce] can)

- Flaxseed

- Matcha green
  tea powder

- Oats, rolled

- Olive oil

- Peanut butter (or
  use homemade,
  page 157)

- Protein powder

- Shredded coconut

- Tahini (¼ cup)

- Vanilla extract

- Whole-wheat bread
  (2 slices)

- Whole-wheat
  pita (4)

- Whole-wheat
  tortillas (4)

PREP AHEAD

To make your week easier, here are some items to prep ahead.

- Prep 6 Perfect Hard-Boiled Eggs (page 156).

- Prep the Rainbow Hummus (page 160). You can choose the original version or mix it up with one of the variations. You'll use this for quick grab 'n' go snacks throughout this week and next.

- You can prep the 5-Minute Guac (page 164) ahead of time or make it day of since it is quick and easy. If prepping ahead, keep the avocado pit and place it in the guacamole before refrigerating it to help keep it from browning.

- Prep the Roasted Chickpeas (page 137). You'll have these available for snacking and as an easy add-in for salads. Use them for the Chickpea and Pear Kale Salad (page 84). You can also add them to the Crunchy Kale and Salmon Salad (page 98) and the Weeknight Steak Salad (page 117) for some added fiber and crunch. You will also use these in Week 2.

- To save a couple minutes, you can always prep some "Dress It Up" Salad Dressing (page 165) ahead of time to keep in your refrigerator. You'll use it on each of the salads for the weekly menus.

- Clean, wash, and prep veggies to help with your meal prep for the week. This will make your smoothies, snacks, and frittata come together in minutes. You can even prep all the ingredients for the smoothies and freeze them until you're ready to pop them into the blender.

- To save time, you can make the Creamy Peanut Butter (page 157) in advance or choose a store-bought brand that's low in additives. You'll use it for snacking and smoothies.

- Prepare the Homemade Pita Chips (page 155).

14-Day Plan for Fat Loss: Week 2

	BREAKFAST	SNACK	LUNCH	SNACK	DINNER	WORKOUT
MONDAY	Sunshine Smoothie (page 44) + additional protein as suggested in tips	Carrots + 2 table-spoons Rainbow Hummus (page 160)	Easy Tuna Niçoise Salad (page 88)	Apple + 2 table-spoons Creamy Peanut Butter (page 157)	Stir-Fry Beef with Vegetables (page 118)	Fat Loss Strength Training Routine #3 (page 172)
TUESDAY	Sunshine Smoothie (leftover)	2 Perfect Hard-Boiled Eggs (page 156)	Stir-Fry Beef with Vegetables (leftover)	Snap peas and cucum-bers + Better-for-You Ranch Dip (page 166)	Sheet-Pan Sweet Potatoes with Crispy Chickpeas (page 69). Can add grilled chicken or fish for additional protein.	Cardio
WEDNESDAY	Fancy Avocado Toast (page 53) + 2 eggs	Apple + 2 table-spoons Creamy Peanut Butter (leftover)	Chickpea and Pear Kale Salad (page 84)	Carrots + 2 table-spoons Rainbow Hummus (leftover)	Oven-Roasted Fish with Burst Tomatoes (page 93)	HIIT

	BREAKFAST	SNACK	LUNCH	SNACK	DINNER	WORKOUT
THURSDAY	Superfood Overnight Oats (page 50)	Snap peas and cucumbers + Better-for-You Ranch Dip (leftover)	Oven-Roasted Fish with Burst Tomatoes (leftover)	2 Perfect Hard-Boiled Eggs (leftover)	Grilled Chicken with Avocado and Tomato Salad (page 105)	Rest + Recover Day
FRIDAY	Superfood Overnight Oats (leftover)	2 Perfect Hard-Boiled Eggs (leftover)	*Leftover grilled chicken from dinner on bed of greens + "Dress It Up" Salad Dressing (page 165)*	Apple + 2 tablespoons Creamy Peanut Butter (leftover)	**READER'S CHOICE**	Fat Loss Strength Training Routine #1 (page 170)
SATURDAY	Goat Cheese and Tomato Breakfast Wraps (page 57)	Snap peas and cucumbers + Better-for-You Ranch Dip (leftover)	Turkey and Veggie Burgers with Sweet Potatoes (page 102)	Carrots + 2 tablespoons Rainbow Hummus (leftover)	**READER'S CHOICE**	Cardio
SUNDAY	**READER'S CHOICE**	2 Perfect Hard-Boiled Eggs (leftover)	Turkey and Veggie Burgers with Sweet Potatoes (leftover)	Apple + 2 tablespoons Creamy Peanut Butter (leftover)	**READER'S CHOICE**	Rest + Recover Day

SHOPPING LIST

PRODUCE

- Apple, green (1)
- Apples, color of choice (4)
- Arugula (1 cup)
- Avocados (3)
- Baby red potatoes (1 cup)
- Banana (1)
- Bell pepper (1)
- Broccoli (½ head)
- Carrots (3)
- Celery (1 stalk)

- Chives, fresh
  (1 bunch)
- Cucumber (1)
- Dill, fresh (1 bunch)
- Garlic (3 cloves)
- Green beans (1 cup)
- Lemons (2)
- Limes (2)
- Mushrooms (¼ cup)
- Parsley, fresh
  (1 bunch)
- Pear (1)
- Scallions (2)
- Snap peas (1 cup)
- Spinach (1 cup)
- Sweet potatoes (2)
- Tomatoes, cherry
  (1 pint)
- Tomatoes,
  heirloom (2)
- Tomato, Roma (1)
- Zucchini (1)

DAIRY AND EGGS

- Eggs, large
  (1 dozen)
- Goat cheese,
  crumbled
  (2 ounces)
- Greek yogurt
  (10 ounces)
- Milk or unsweet-
  ened nondairy
  alternative
  (10 ounces)

MEAT AND SEAFOOD

- Chicken breasts,
  boneless,
  skinless (2)
- Cod, salmon,
  or halibut fillets
  (12 ounces)
- Stir-fry steak
  (8 ounces)
- Tuna (1 [5-ounce]
  can)
- Turkey, ground
  (8 ounces)

FROZEN

- Blueberries (½ cup;
  can buy fresh
  instead)
- Corn kernels
  (½ cup)
- Peach slices (½ cup;
  can buy fresh
  instead)
- Pineapple (½ cup;
  can buy fresh
  instead)

HERBS AND SPICES

- Black pepper
- Cayenne pepper
- Cinnamon, ground
- Garlic powder
- Ginger (ground; can buy fresh instead)
- Onion powder
- Paprika
- Red pepper flakes
- Salt

PANTRY

- Chia seeds
- Chickpeas (2 [15-ounce] cans)
- Cornstarch
- Flaxseed
- Honey
- Matcha green tea powder
- Oats, rolled
- Olives, Kalamata, pitted
- Olive oil
- Peanut butter (or use homemade, page 157)
- Sesame oil
- Soy sauce
- Vanilla extract
- Walnuts
- Whole-grain bread (2 slices)
- Whole-grain hamburger buns (2)
- Whole-grain pita (2)
- Whole-grain tortillas (2)

PREP AHEAD

To make your week easier, here are some items to prep ahead.

- Prep 8 Perfect Hard-Boiled Eggs (page 156).

- Prep "Dress It Up" Salad Dressing (page 165) ahead of time and keep in your refrigerator.

- Prep a batch of Better-for-You Ranch Dip (page 166). You will use this for snacking.

- Clean, wash, and prep veggies to speed up meal prep for the week. You can also prep all the ingredients for smoothies and freeze them until you're ready to pop them into the blender.

- To save time, you can make Creamy Peanut Butter (page 157) in advance or choose a store-bought brand that's low in additives.

14-Day Plan for Muscle Gain: Week 1

	BREAKFAST	SNACK	LUNCH	SNACK	DINNER	WORKOUT
MONDAY	Banana-Nut Smoothie (page 48)	Almond Butter Protein Bites (page 139) + 7 ounces Greek yogurt	Tuna Power Wraps (page 90)	Banana-Nut Smoothie (leftover)	Chili-Rubbed Steak Tacos (page 116) + 5-Minute Guac (page 164)	Muscle Gain Strength Training Routine #1 (page 174)
TUESDAY	Superfood Overnight Oats (page 50) + protein powder	Almond Butter Protein Bites (leftover) + 7 ounces Greek yogurt	Weeknight Steak Salad (page 117) *(using leftover steak from dinner)* + 1 slice whole-grain bread for additional carbs	2 Perfect Hard-Boiled Eggs (page 156) + 1 small apple	Orzo with Broccoli and Pine Nuts (page 66). Can add grilled chicken or steak for additional protein.	HIIT
WEDNESDAY	Superfood Overnight Oats + protein powder (leftover)	Almond Butter Protein Bites (leftover) + 7 ounces Greek yogurt	Orzo and Arugula Salad (page 72) *(using leftover orzo + protein from dinner)*	Apple + Dessert Hummus (page 143) + 1 Perfect Hard-Boiled Egg (leftover)	Easy Breaded Pork Chops (page 124)	Rest + Recover Day
THURSDAY	On-the-Go Tropical Breakfast Bowls (page 49) (halve to make only one serving). To minimize fat, can omit coconut. For additional protein, can increase Greek yogurt.	2 Perfect Hard-Boiled Eggs (leftover)	Easy Breaded Pork Chops (leftover) + fresh green salad	Stuffed Avocado (page 138)	Sheet-Pan Sausage and Brussels Sprouts (page 122) using lean sausage. Can add 1 slice whole-grain bread for additional carbs.	Muscle Gain Strength Training Routine #2 (page 175)

	BREAKFAST	SNACK	LUNCH	SNACK	DINNER	WORKOUT
FRIDAY	Butternut Squash Breakfast Hash (page 58)	½ cup Perfect Granola (leftover) + 7 ounces Greek yogurt	Sheet-Pan Sausage and Brussels Sprouts (leftover) + store-bought sauerkraut and mustard	Apple + Dessert Hummus (leftover)	**READER'S CHOICE**	HIIT
SATURDAY	**READER'S CHOICE**	Blueberry–Peanut Butter Muffins (page 141) + 7 ounces Greek yogurt	Cauliflower Tacos with Avocado Crema (page 68) Can add black beans for additional fiber and protein.	Rainbow Hummus (leftover) + Homemade Pita Chips (page 155) and veggies	**READER'S CHOICE**	Cardio
SUNDAY	Powered-Up Pancakes (page 54) + 2 poached eggs	Blueberry–Peanut Butter Muffins (leftover)	**READER'S CHOICE**	Rainbow Hummus (leftover) + Homemade Pita Chips (leftover) and veggies	Shrimp Scampi with Whole-Grain Pasta (page 94)	Rest + Recover Day

SHOPPING LIST

PRODUCE

- Alfalfa sprouts (½ cup)
- Apples (4)
- Arugula (1 cup)
- Avocado (1)
- Banana (1)
- Broccoli (2 cups)
- Brussels sprouts (1 pound)
- Butternut squash (1 small)
- Cabbage, red (¼ small head)
- Cauliflower (1 small head)
- Celery (2 stalks)
- Garlic (2 cloves)
- Limes (2)
- Lemons (3)
- Onion (1)
- Spinach (4½ cups)
- Tomatoes, cherry (1 cup)
- Tomato (1)
- Zucchini (1)

DAIRY AND EGGS

- Blue cheese, crumbled (1 ounce; optional)
- Eggs, large (15)
- Greek yogurt (56 ounces)
- Milk or unsweetened nondairy alternative (20 ounces)
- Mozzarella cheese (¼ cup)
- Parmesan cheese (2 ounces)

MEAT AND SEAFOOD

- Bratwurst or Italian sausage (8 ounces)
- Chicken breast (2)
- Flank steak (1¼ pounds)
- Pork chops, bone-in (2)
- Shrimp (6 ounces)
- Tuna (1 can)
- Turkey, ground (4 ounces)

FROZEN

- Blueberries (1½ cups; can buy fresh instead)

HERBS AND SPICES

- Basil, dried
- Black pepper
- Chili powder
- Cinnamon, ground
- Cumin, ground
- Garlic powder
- Italian seasoning
- Onion powder
- Oregano, dried
- Paprika
- Red pepper flakes
- Sage, dried
- Salt
- Thyme, dried

PANTRY

- Applesauce (¼ cup)
- Brown sugar
- Chia seeds
- Chickpeas (2 [15-ounce] cans)
- Cocoa powder
- Coconut oil
- Dark chocolate chips
- Dates, pitted

- Dried tart cherries
- Flaxseed
- Honey
- Maple syrup, pure
- Mustard, whole-grain
- Oats, rolled
- Oat flour
- Olive oil
- Orzo (1 cup)

- Peanut butter (or use homemade, page 157)
- Pine nuts
- Protein powder
- Sauerkraut
- Shredded coconut
- Sun-dried tomatoes
- Walnuts
- Whole-grain bread (2 slices)

- Whole-grain linguine or spaghetti
- Whole-grain pita (2)
- Whole-grain tortillas (6)
- Whole-wheat panko breadcrumbs

PREP AHEAD

To make your week easier, here are some items to prep ahead.

- Prep 5 Perfect Hard-Boiled Eggs (page 156).

- Prep 1 cup of Rainbow Hummus (page 160) and Homemade Pita Chips (page 155). You can choose the original version or mix it up with one of the variations.

- Prep Dessert Hummus (page 143) to have available as a sweet post-workout snack.

- To save a couple minutes, you can always prep some "Dress It Up" Salad Dressing (page 165) ahead of time and keep in your refrigerator.

- Clean, wash, and cut veggies to speed up meal prep for the week and to pair with your hummus and pita for snacks.

- You can prep all ingredients for smoothies and freeze them until you're ready to pop them into the blender.

- Make Perfect Granola (page 154). You can pair this with Greek yogurt for a quick snack for the next couple of weeks.

- Prep Almond Butter Protein Bites (page 139)—you'll have these as a snack for the next two weeks.

- Prep Blueberry–Peanut Butter Muffins (page 141)—you'll have these as a snack for the next two weeks.

14-Day Plan for Muscle Gain: Week 2

	BREAKFAST	SNACK	LUNCH	SNACK	DINNER	WORKOUT
MONDAY	Berry Berry Breakfast Quinoa (page 52) + 1 Perfect Hard-Boiled Egg (page 156)	Almond Butter Protein Bites (leftover) + 7 ounces Greek yogurt	Tuna Power Wraps (page 90) + piece of fruit	Stuffed Avocado (page 138)	Lamb Meatballs with Yogurt (page 130). Can add rice or other grain for additional carbs.	Muscle Gain Strength Training Routine #3 (page 176)
TUESDAY	Berry Berry Breakfast Quinoa (leftover)	½ cup Perfect Granola (page 154) + 7 ounces Greek yogurt	Spiced Lamb, Brown Rice, and Hummus Bowls (*using leftover lamb meatballs from dinner*)	2 Perfect Hard-Boiled Eggs (leftover)	Sweet and Savory Grilled Pork Chops (page 123). Can add rice + steamed veggies for additional carbs.	HIIT
WEDNESDAY	Fancy Avocado Toast (page 53) + 2 eggs	Almond Butter Protein Bites (leftover) + 7 ounces Greek yogurt	Sweet and Savory Grilled Pork Chops (leftover)	Stuffed Avocado (leftover)	Chickpea and Couscous Salad (page 70) + 3 ounces grilled chicken, steak, or salmon.	Rest + Recover Day
THURSDAY	On-the-Go Tropical Breakfast Bowls (page 49)	2 Perfect Hard-Boiled Eggs (leftover)	Chickpea and Couscous Salad (leftover)	Apple + Dessert Hummus (page 143)	One-Pan Steak and Potatoes (page 119)	Muscle Gain Strength Training Routine #1 (page 174)

	BREAKFAST	SNACK	LUNCH	SNACK	DINNER	WORKOUT
FRIDAY	On-the-Go Tropical Breakfast Bowls (leftover)	½ cup berries + 7 ounces Greek yogurt	*Leftover steak from dinner + salad*	Apple + Dessert Hummus (leftover)	**READER'S CHOICE**	HIIT
SATURDAY	Veggie-Ful Egg Bake (page 60)	Blueberry– Peanut Butter Muffins (leftover) + 7 ounces Greek yogurt	Beef Nacho'd Peppers (page 115)	2 Perfect Hard-Boiled Eggs (leftover)	**READER'S CHOICE**	Cardio
SUNDAY	**READER'S CHOICE**	Blueberry– Peanut Butter Muffins (leftover)	**READER'S CHOICE**	Almond Butter Protein Bites (leftover)	Mediterranean Lamb Flatbreads (page 126)	Rest + Recover Day

SHOPPING LIST

PRODUCE

- Alfalfa sprouts (½ cup)

- Apples (3)

- Asparagus (1 bunch)

- Avocados (3)

- Baby red potatoes (½ pound)

- Bananas (2)

- Bell pepper (1)

- Bell peppers, mini (½ bag)

- Berries (½ cup)

- Celery (2 stalks)

- Cucumbers (2)

- Garlic (4 cloves)

- Ginger, fresh (1)

- Jalapeño (1)

- Lemons (2)

- Lime (1)

- Mangos (2)

- Mint, fresh (1 bunch)

- Onions, red (2)

- Onion, yellow (1)

- Romaine lettuce (2 cups)

- Rosemary, fresh (1 sprig)

- Spinach (1½ cups)
- Tomatoes (3)
- Tomatoes, cherry (10 ounces)

DAIRY AND EGGS

- Eggs, large (14)
- Feta cheese, crumbled (2 ounces)
- Goat cheese, crumbled (1 ounce)
- Greek yogurt (49 ounces)
- Mexican cheese, shredded (½ cup)
- Milk or unsweetened nondairy alternative (14 ounces)

MEAT AND SEAFOOD

- Beef, lean ground (8 ounce)
- Chicken breast (1)
- Lamb, ground (1½ pounds)
- Pork chops, boneless (2)
- Skirt steak (8 ounces)
- Tuna (1 [5-ounce] can)

FROZEN

- Berries of choice (¼ cup; can buy fresh instead)

HERBS AND SPICES

- Allspice, ground
- Basil, dried
- Black pepper
- Cayenne pepper
- Chili powder
- Cinnamon, ground
- Cumin, ground
- Garlic powder
- Minced onion
- Oregano, dried
- Parsley, dried
- Red pepper flakes
- Salt

PANTRY

- Black beans (1 [15-ounce] can)
- Brown rice
- Chia seeds
- Chickpeas (2 [15-ounce] cans)
- Couscous
- Flaxseed

- Green chiles (1 [4-ounce] can)
- Mustard, whole-grain
- Oats, rolled
- Olives, Kalamata
- Olive oil
- Peanut butter (or use homemade, page 157)

- Pesto (or use homemade, page 158)
- Protein powder
- Quinoa
- Vinegar, balsamic
- Vinegar, red wine
- Walnuts

- Whole-grain bread (2 slices)
- Whole-wheat naan (2)
- Whole-wheat pita (2)
- Whole-wheat tortillas (2)

PREP AHEAD

To make your week easier, here are some items to prep ahead.

- Prep 7 Perfect Hard-Boiled Eggs (page 156).

- To save a couple minutes, you can always prep some "Dress It Up" Salad Dressing ahead of time and keep in your refrigerator. You will use it on each of the salads for the week.

- Clean, wash, and cut veggies to speed up meal prep for the week.

- You can prep all ingredients for the smoothies and freeze them until you're ready to pop them into the blender.

- If you need to save time, you can purchase pesto. If you prefer to make it at home, you can try Macro-Friendly Pesto (page 158).

- Prep the quinoa, couscous, and brown rice for the week and store each in an airtight container.

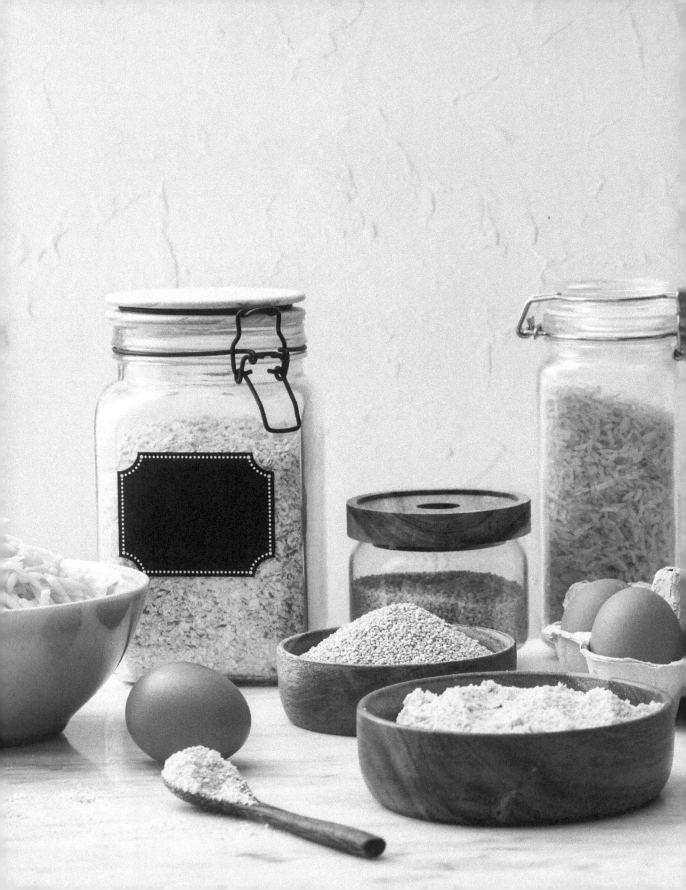

PART TWO
THE RECIPES

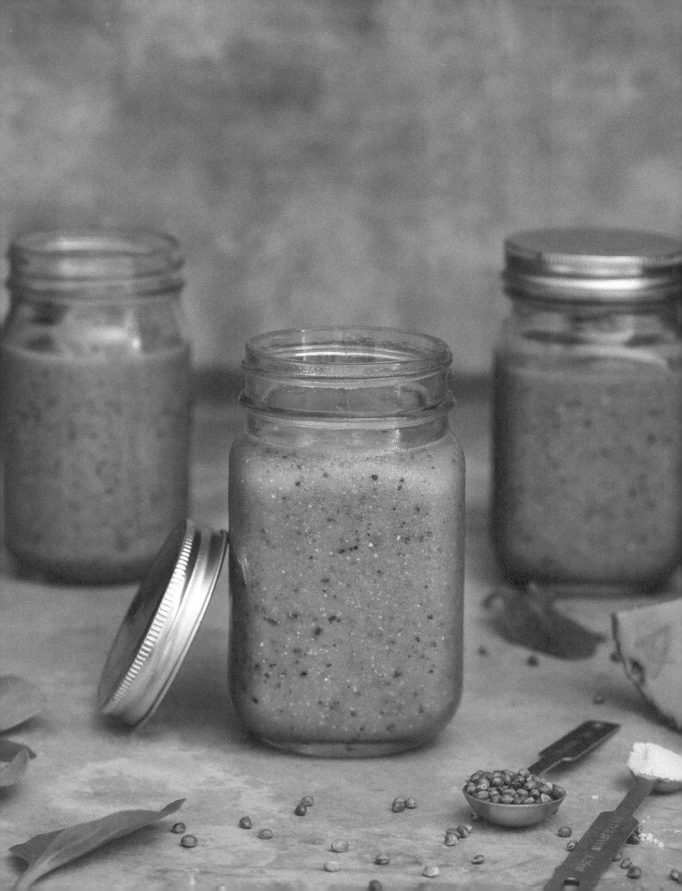

3

BREAKFASTS

Sunshine Smoothie

PREP TIME: 5 minutes • **SERVES 2**

A smoothie is a quick and easy way to get in your greens, fruits, fiber, and protein. Adding ground flaxseed increases these benefits while adding vitamins and minerals, including thiamin (vitamin B$_1$), magnesium, and phosphorus, as well as omega-3 fatty acids. By adding just 1 tablespoon of ground flaxseed, you'll add 1.5 grams of protein, 2 grams of fiber, and 2.5 grams of unsaturated fats to your smoothie.

1 cup fresh or frozen peach slices

½ cup blueberries

1 banana

1 cup spinach

2 cups 1% milk or unsweetened nondairy alternative

2 tablespoons Creamy Peanut Butter (page 157) or store-bought

1 tablespoon ground flaxseed

¾ cup ice

1. Combine the peach, blueberries, banana, spinach, milk, peanut butter, flaxseed, and ice in a blender and blend or pulse until smooth. If using frozen fruit, you may not need as much ice.

2. Serve immediately and enjoy!

MUSCLE GAIN: To increase the total protein, protein powders blend in nicely and are made from a variety of protein sources, such as dairy-based (whey or casein), nondairy (soy, pea, or rice), and bovine-based collagen. Speak with your dietitian or healthcare provider to find the best one for you.

You could also add hemp seeds (3 tablespoons contain 10 grams of protein) or plain Greek yogurt (7 ounces for 20 grams of high-quality protein).

PER SERVING (ABOUT 12 FL OZ): Calories: 323; Protein: 14g; Total Carbohydrates: 42g; Fiber: 6g; Fat: 13g

MACROS: 17% Protein; 33% Fat; 50% Carbohydrates

Eat-Your-Greens Smoothie

PREP TIME: 5 minutes • **SERVES 2**

Delicious pineapple is packed with nutrients, antioxidants, and enzymes that naturally help fight against inflammation and disease, and it helps balance out the greens in this smoothie with its sweet-tart flavor. The avocado provides healthy omega-3s while enhancing the creaminess you'll love. After a workout, you can swap out the milk for coconut water to help you replenish electrolytes and rehydrate.

2 cups spinach or kale

1 cup cubed fresh or frozen
  pineapple

1 green apple, cored

2 celery stalks, chunked

½ avocado

2 cups 1% milk or unsweetened
  nondairy alternative

1 cup ice

1. Combine the spinach, pineapple, apple, celery, avocado, milk, and ice in a blender and blend or pulse until smooth. If using frozen fruit, you may not need as much ice.

2. Serve immediately and enjoy!

MUSCLE GAIN: Explore ways to add protein, whether through protein powder, plain Greek yogurt, or nut butter. A little goes a long way in helping you meet your daily goals.

PER SERVING (ABOUT 12 FL OZ): Calories: 285; Protein: 11g; Total Carbohydrates: 42g; Fiber: 8g; Fat: 10g

MACROS: 15% Protein; 30% Fat; 55% Carbohydrates

Chia-Matcha Smoothie Bowls

PREP TIME: 10 minutes • **SERVES 2**

Chia seeds may be small, but they're big on nutrition. Just 1 ounce of this superfood contains 5 grams of protein, 9 grams of fat (an excellent source of omega-3s), 10 grams of fiber, and a variety of antioxidants, as well as calcium, iron, magnesium, phosphorus, and zinc. To top it off, they'll also help thicken your smoothie to the perfect consistency.

2 tablespoons chia seeds, plus 2 teaspoons for topping

2 cups unsweetened almond milk

¼ cup rolled oats (not instant)

½ cup spinach

2 large bananas

2 teaspoons matcha green tea powder

1 teaspoon vanilla extract

½ cup ice

½ cup mixed berries, for topping

½ banana, sliced, for topping

1 tablespoon shredded coconut, for topping

1. In a small bowl, combine the chia seeds and almond milk. Set aside for 10 minutes.

2. While the chia seeds are soaking, put the oats in a high-speed blender and pulse until finely ground.

3. Add the chia mixture, spinach, bananas, matcha, vanilla, and ice to the blender with the oats. Blend until smooth.

4. Divide the smoothie between two bowls and evenly add the toppings to each bowl. Serve immediately.

MUSCLE GAIN: To bump up the protein, swap out the almond milk for 1 cup of plain Greek yogurt.

PER SERVING (ABOUT 12 FL OZ): Calories: 390; Protein: 15g; Total Carbohydrates: 69g; Fiber: 13g; Fat: 7g

MACROS: 15% Protein; 16% Fat; 69% Carbohydrates

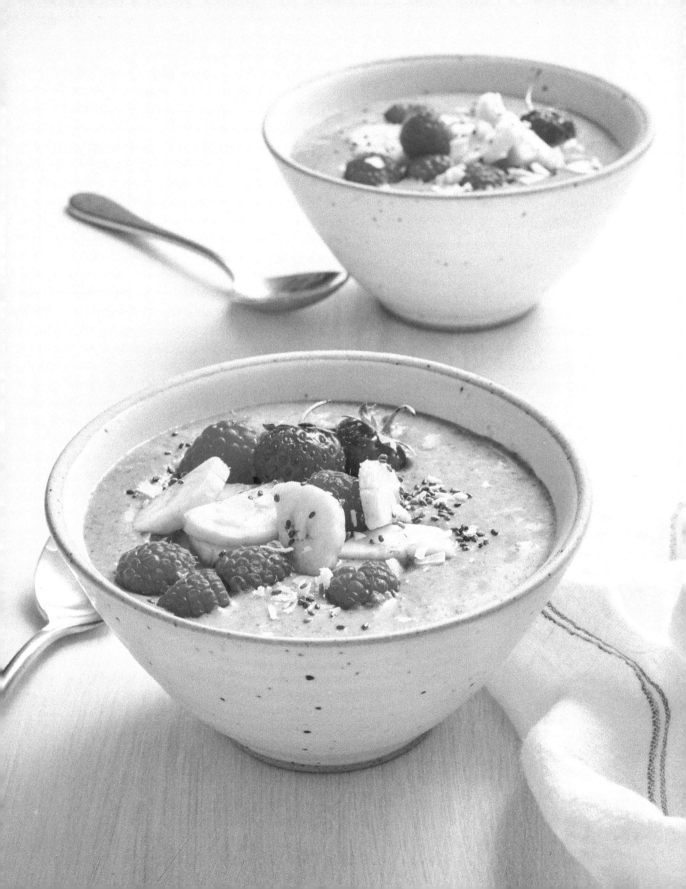

Banana-Nut Smoothie

PREP TIME: 5 minutes • **SERVES 2**

Banana bread is a comfort food to many, so why not make it into a smoothie? Bananas are a great source of vitamin A, vitamin C, vitamin B$_6$, potassium, and magnesium. Add walnuts and chia seeds to that equation and you have a powerhouse of a meal that can be enjoyed in the comfort of your home or on the go.

1 banana

2 tablespoons Creamy Peanut Butter (page 157) or store-bought

2 cups 1% milk or unsweetened nondairy alternative

2 tablespoons chia seeds

½ teaspoon ground cinnamon

1 cup ice

1 scoop vanilla or unflavored protein powder

½ cup chopped walnuts or granola, for garnish (optional)

1. Combine the banana, peanut butter, milk, chia seeds, cinnamon, ice, and protein powder in a blender and blend or pulse until smooth.

2. Top with chopped walnuts or granola, if desired.

3. Serve immediately and enjoy!

FAT LOSS: Fiber and fat both aid in helping us feel fuller for a longer. To convert this to a fat loss recipe, add 1 cup of spinach (4 grams of fiber) or 1 cup of canned pumpkin (7 grams of fiber).

PER SERVING (ABOUT 12 FL OZ): Calories: 409; Protein: 27g; Total Carbohydrates: 42g; Fiber: 9g; Fat: 16g

MACROS: 26% Protein; 34% Fat; 40% Carbohydrates

On-the-Go Tropical Breakfast Bowls

PREP TIME: 5 minutes • **SERVES 2**

Greek yogurt is an incredibly versatile ingredient and typically has a higher protein content that other types of yogurt. A 7-ounce portion boasts 20 grams of protein and is particularly rich in vitamin B$_{12}$, riboflavin, and selenium.

2 cups plain low- or nonfat Greek yogurt
½ cup Perfect Granola (page 154) or store-bought
1 large banana, sliced
2 tablespoons chia seeds
½ cup shredded coconut

1. Scoop 1 cup of yogurt into each of two bowls.

2. Divide the granola equally between the bowls on top of the yogurt.

3. Finish topping each bowl with ½ banana, 1 tablespoon of chia, and ¼ cup of coconut.

4. Enjoy immediately.

FAT LOSS: To cut carbs, choose granola that's heavier on seeds and nuts instead of grains and consider cutting the portions of other ingredients, such as using ½ banana instead of a full one. It's also critical to use plain Greek yogurt rather than ones with added sugars or sweeteners.

PER SERVING (ABOUT 8 OZ): Calories: 499; Protein: 18g; Total Carbohydrates: 52g; Fiber: 11g; Fat: 26g

MACROS: 14% Protein; 46% Fat; 40% Carbohydrates

Superfood Overnight Oats

PREP TIME: 5 minutes (plus overnight to soak) • **SERVES 2**

Packed with superfood ingredients, these overnight oats will give you the head start you've been looking for. Oats are a whole-grain food that's packed with nutrients. They're a great source of complex carbohydrates, protein, and fiber, delivering a balanced blood sugar response when added to breakfast, muffins, cookies, or dessert!

2 cups rolled oats (not instant)

2 cups 1% milk or unsweetened nondairy alternative

1 tablespoon ground flaxseed

½ cup chopped walnuts

1 cup fresh or frozen blueberries

1 tablespoon honey

1 teaspoon ground cinnamon

1. Combine the oats, milk, flaxseed, walnuts, blueberries, honey, and cinnamon in a bowl or large mason jar.

2. Stir or shake until all ingredients are well mixed together.

3. Cover and place in your refrigerator overnight.

4. In the morning, uncover and enjoy!

5. If the consistency is a bit thicker than you'd like, you're welcome to add more milk until your desired consistency is achieved.

MUSCLE GAIN: Adding 2 scoops of unflavored protein or collagen powder will provide 20 more grams of protein, a morning boost to help you hit your protein macro goal for the day. If looking to cut down on sweetness, you can always leave out the honey.

PER SERVING (ABOUT 8 OZ): Calories: 540; Protein: 22g; Total Carbohydrates: 63g; Fiber: 10g; Fat: 25g

MACROS: 14% Protein; 35% Fat; 51% Carbohydrates

PB&B Overnight Oats

PREP TIME: 5 minutes (plus overnight to soak) • **SERVES 2**

Peanut butter is one of the world's most popular spreads (and if you're anything like me, it's one of your favorites). If you shop for it rather than making your own, look for peanut butter that's relatively unprocessed—basically roasted peanuts and maybe a bit of salt. Watch out for added sugar, trans fats, and vegetable oils.

1 banana

2 tablespoons Creamy Peanut Butter (page 157) or store-bought

½ cup plain low- or nonfat Greek yogurt

½ cup 1% milk or unsweetened nondairy alternative

1 teaspoon vanilla extract

1 cup rolled oats (not instant)

1 tablespoon ground flaxseed

1 teaspoon ground cinnamon

1. In a large bowl, mash the banana.

2. Add the peanut butter, yogurt, milk, and vanilla. Mix until smooth and well blended.

3. Add the oats, flaxseed, and cinnamon. Stir to combine.

4. You can keep the mixture in the bowl or divide it between two mason jars.

5. Cover and refrigerate overnight.

6. In the morning, uncover and enjoy!

MUSCLE GAIN: Add 2 scoops of protein or collagen powder for 20 grams of additional protein. You can also increase the total amount of Greek yogurt and/or milk to provide a bump in protein and carbohydrates, helping you meet your daily goals.

PER SERVING (ABOUT 10 OZ): Calories: 327; Protein: 12g; Total Carbohydrates: 37g; Fiber: 15g; Fat: 15g

MACROS: 14% Protein; 40% Fat; 46% Carbohydrates

Berry Berry Breakfast Quinoa

PREP TIME: 10 minutes • **COOK TIME:** 30 minutes • **SERVES 2**

Quinoa is gaining more and more popularity here in the United States, though South America has been cultivating it since ancient times. It's gluten-free and nourishing, delivering 8 grams of protein and 5 grams of fiber in just a single cup, along with nutrients including folate, copper, iron, zinc, manganese, magnesium, and phosphorus.

1 cup quinoa

2 cups water

¼ teaspoon salt

1 cup 1% milk or unsweetened nondairy alternative

1 teaspoon ground cinnamon

1 teaspoon vanilla extract

1 banana, sliced

½ cup blueberries or berry of choice

2 tablespoons nut butter, such as Creamy Peanut Butter (page 157)

2 tablespoons chopped walnuts

1 tablespoon ground flaxseed

FAT LOSS: To cut back on carbs, you can use only berries and skip the banana. The berries have a lower glycemic effect and high fiber content, leading to a much more gradual rise in blood sugar.

1. Put the quinoa in a colander and rinse under running water for at least 30 seconds. Drain well.

2. Transfer the rinsed quinoa to a saucepan and add the water and salt.

3. Bring the mixture to a boil over medium-high heat, uncovered. Once boiling, reduce to a simmer. Cook until the quinoa has absorbed all the water, 15 to 20 minutes.

4. Remove the pan from the heat, cover, and let rest for 5 minutes.

5. After the quinoa has rested, add the milk, cinnamon, and vanilla. Stir over medium heat until mixed and heated through.

6. Divide the quinoa between two bowls and top each with the banana, blueberries, nut butter, walnuts, and flaxseed.

7. Enjoy immediately or store in the refrigerator for up to 2 days.

PER SERVING (ABOUT 12 OZ): Calories: 615; Protein: 22g; Total Carbohydrates: 85g; Fiber: 12g; Fat: 23g

MACROS: 14% Protein; 31% Fat; 55% Carbohydrates

Fancy Avocado Toast

PREP TIME: 10 minutes • **SERVES 2**

Avocado toast has made its way to breakfast menus all over the world, and for good reason. Avocados are satisfying, contain unsaturated fats that have been found to lower LDL cholesterol, and deliver more potassium per gram than bananas. They're also an excellent source of fiber and folate, making them a fan-favorite.

2 ripe avocados
Juice of 1 lemon
Flaky sea salt
4 slices whole-grain bread, toasted
Everything bagel seasoning, for topping (optional)

1. Cut the avocados in half and remove the pits.

2. Using a small knife, dice the avocado flesh while it's still in the skin. Sprinkle with the lemon juice and salt.

3. Scoop the diced avocado out of the skin and onto the toasted bread, dividing it evenly among the slices.

4. Mash the avocado with the back of a fork and top with everything bagel seasoning, if desired.

MUSCLE GAIN: Adding a cooked egg on top of your avocado toast will provide you with an additional 6 grams of protein, helping you meet your muscle-gain goal. A single egg also adds 5 grams of healthy fats, as well as vitamins D, E, K, and B_6 and calcium, zinc, choline, selenium, and folate.

PER SERVING (2 SLICES): Calories: 367; Protein: 5g; Total Carbohydrates: 26g; Fiber: 12g; Fat: 27g

MACROS: 6% Protein; 66% Fat; 28% Carbohydrates

Powered-Up Pancakes

PREP TIME: 10 minutes • **COOK TIME:** 10 minutes • **SERVES 4**

Adding unsweetened applesauce to any recipe is a great option when you're looking to cut back on oils and saturated fats, as it helps retain moisture. This recipe takes your typical pancake and turns it up a notch with some added protein and fiber, and less total sugar overall. And if it fits your macros, feel free to top with berries and maple syrup.

½ cup 1% milk or unsweetened nondairy alternative

3 large eggs

½ cup plain low- or nonfat Greek yogurt

½ cup unsweetened applesauce

½ teaspoon vanilla extract

1 tablespoon unsalted butter or coconut oil, melted and cooled

1½ cups rolled oats (not instant)

½ teaspoon ground cinnamon

Oil, for greasing the pan

1. In a large bowl, whisk together the milk, eggs, yogurt, applesauce, vanilla, and cooled butter.

2. Add the oats and cinnamon and mix until incorporated. Let stand for 5 minutes.

3. Grease a griddle or pan with oil and heat over medium heat. Once the pan is ready, pour batter ⅓ cup at a time into the pan. Cook until bubbles begin to form, then flip and cook the other side.

4. Serve immediately. Leftover pancakes can be stored in an airtight container in the refrigerator for up to 3 days or in the freezer for up to 3 months.

FAT LOSS: Focus on adding fiber to help with satiety. You can sprinkle the pancakes with flaxseed and cinnamon once cooked, or you can add 1 tablespoon of flaxseed straight into the batter.

PER SERVING (2 PANCAKES): Calories: 243; Protein: 12g; Total Carbohydrates: 26g; Fiber: 4g; Fat: 10g

MACROS: 19% Protein; 37% Fat; 44% Carbohydrates

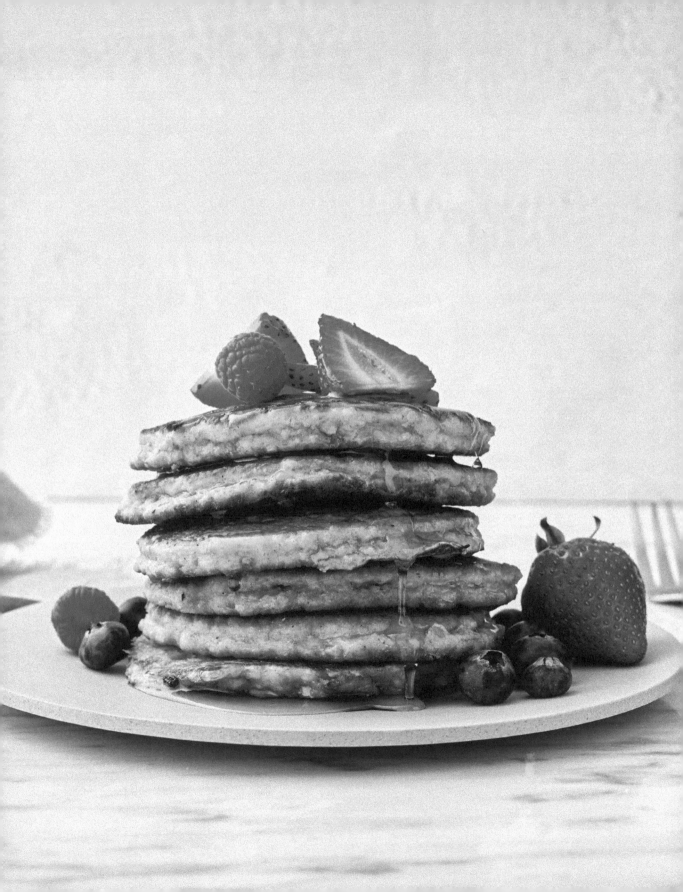

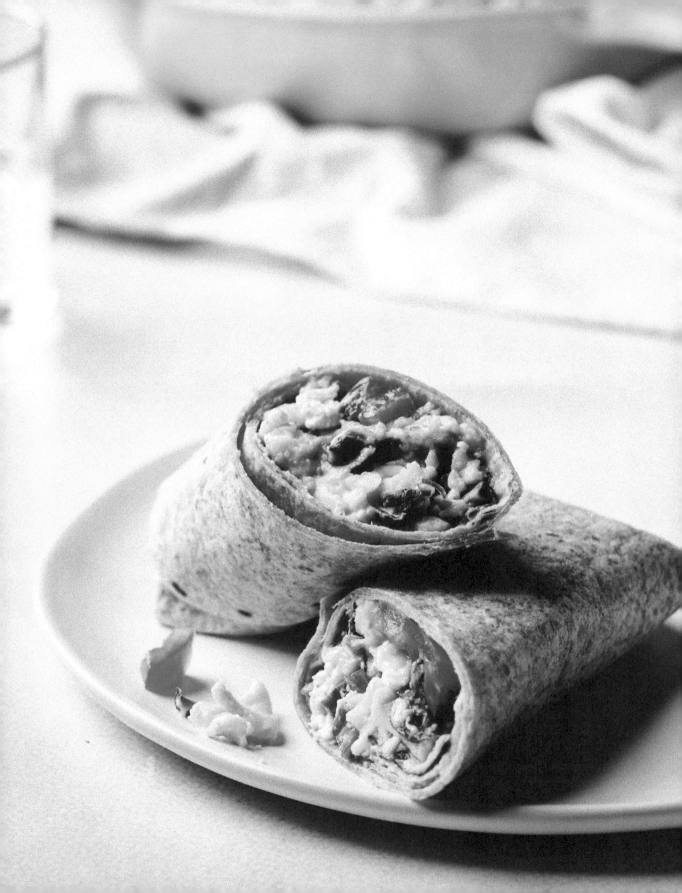

Goat Cheese and Tomato Breakfast Wraps

PREP TIME: 10 minutes • **COOK TIME:** 10 minutes • **SERVES 4**

Vegetables for breakfast? Yes! Every meal is an opportunity to get vegetables in. You can easily add more to these wraps, like mushrooms or bell peppers, to increase the phytonutrient load and volume of the meal. Remember, eat the rainbow!

4 large eggs

⅓ cup 1% milk or unsweetened nondairy alternative

¼ teaspoon freshly ground black pepper

¼ teaspoon salt

1 tablespoon olive oil

4 cups baby spinach

¼ cup crumbled goat cheese

2 scallions, green parts only, finely chopped

4 large whole-wheat tortillas

1 Roma tomato, diced

MUSCLE GAIN: To increase the protein load, double the amount of egg included, taking this to 8 eggs total for 4 servings. This would take the amount of protein up to 19 grams per wrap, while only raising the total fat by 5 grams.

1. In a medium bowl, whisk together the eggs, milk, pepper, and salt. Set aside.

2. In a large skillet, heat the olive oil over medium heat. Add the spinach and cook until it starts to wilt, about 1 minute.

3. Pour the egg mixture into the skillet and cook until the eggs begin to set, about 2 minutes. Using a wooden spoon, gently stir the eggs, forming large curds, and cook until the eggs are completely set, 2 to 3 minutes. Remove from the heat, add the goat cheese and scallions, and stir to combine.

4. To assemble the wraps: Spoon equal amounts of scrambled egg into the middle of each of the tortillas. Top with diced tomato. Fold in the sides of the tortillas and roll into a wrap.

PER SERVING (1 WRAP): Calories: 245; Protein: 13g; Total Carbohydrates: 27g; Fiber: 5g; Fat: 10g

MACROS: 21% Protein; 36% Fat; 43% Carbohydrates

Butternut Squash Breakfast Hash

PREP TIME: 10 minutes • **COOK TIME:** 15 minutes • **SERVES 4**

This dish takes on the flavors of traditional breakfast sausage like garlic, sage, and thyme, but without the excess saturated fats. The butternut squash complements the flavors well, creating a filling, savory breakfast.

2 tablespoons extra-virgin olive oil, divided

½ onion, diced

1 small butternut squash, peeled, seeded, and cut into ¼-inch dice

8 ounces ground turkey

½ teaspoon garlic powder

1 teaspoon Italian seasoning

¼ teaspoon salt

⅛ teaspoon freshly ground black pepper

3 cups spinach

2 tablespoons maple syrup, for serving

4 teaspoons Sriracha-Style Chile Sauce (page 162) or store-bought, for serving (optional)

1. In a large sauté pan, heat 1 tablespoon of olive oil over medium heat. Add the onion and sauté for about 3 minutes, or until translucent. Add the butternut squash and sauté for about 7 minutes, or until soft.

2. While the butternut squash is cooking, heat the remaining 1 tablespoon of olive oil over medium heat in a separate sauté pan. Add the ground turkey, garlic powder, Italian seasoning, salt, and pepper. Sauté, breaking the turkey up with a spatula, for about 8 minutes, or until browned.

3. When the vegetables are cooked through, add them to the pan with the turkey. Add the spinach and stir to combine.

4. Serve immediately with maple syrup and chile sauce, if desired.

FAT LOSS: For this recipe, the carbs are mainly coming from the squash and maple syrup. An easy adjustment would be to omit the maple syrup to keep this dish ultra-savory and protein heavy.

PER SERVING (ABOUT 1 CUP): Calories: 262; Protein: 16g; Total Carbohydrates: 18g; Fiber: 3g; Fat: 14g

MACROS: 24% Protein; 49% Fat; 27% Carbohydrates

Summer Veggie Frittata

PREP TIME: 10 minutes • **COOK TIME:** 1 hour • **SERVES 4**

The cherry tomatoes add a refreshing touch to this rich frittata. An excellent source of vitamin C and lycopene, these small but mighty vegetables bring an array of health benefits to kick off the day.

Unsalted butter, for greasing the pan

4 slices bacon, cut into 1-inch pieces

2 tablespoons olive oil

1 shallot, thinly sliced

1 medium zucchini, thinly sliced

6 large eggs

½ cup heavy (whipping) cream

1 cup 1% milk or unsweetened nondairy alternative

1 cup cherry tomatoes, cut in half

¾ cup crumbled goat cheese

Salt

Freshly ground black pepper

FAT LOSS: Fiber helps you feel fuller longer, especially when paired with both fats and protein. Serve this frittata with a whole-wheat tortilla or a slice of whole-wheat toast for an added fiber punch.

1. Preheat the oven to 425°F. Grease a 9-inch quiche or pie pan with butter.

2. In a large skillet over medium heat, add bacon and sauté until crispy. Remove from pan and place on a paper towel to absorb grease.

3. Place the skillet with the bacon grease back over medium heat. Add the shallot and sauté, stirring occasionally, until caramelized, 15 to 20 minutes. Add the zucchini, stir to combine, and sauté for another 5 minutes.

4. While the veggies are cooking, whisk together the eggs, cream, and milk in a medium bowl. Set aside.

5. Transfer the shallot and zucchini mixture to the prepared quiche dish. Add the bacon, tomatoes, and goat cheese. Pour in the egg mixture and season with salt and pepper.

6. Bake until the top is golden and the egg mixture looks to be set in the middle, 25 to 30 minutes. Let the frittata cool slightly, then serve by cutting into four wedges.

PER SERVING (1 SLICE): Calories: 436; Protein: 21g; Total Carbohydrates: 9g; Fiber: 1g; Fat: 35g

MACROS: 19% Protein; 72% Fat; 9% Carbohydrates

Veggie-Ful Egg Bake

PREP TIME: 10 minutes • **COOK TIME:** 40 minutes • **SERVES 4**

Vegetables are an easy way to make a meal high in fiber and phytonutrients. Any veggie works for this dish. I love the ones below, but feel free to mix it up with squash, tomatoes, onions, or mushrooms.

Unsalted butter, for greasing
  the pan
1 tablespoon olive oil
1 cup chopped bell pepper, any
  color (about 1 medium)
½ cup thinly sliced scallion
3 cups chopped spinach
6 large eggs
3 tablespoons plain low- or
  nonfat Greek yogurt
½ teaspoon salt
½ teaspoon freshly ground
  black pepper
½ cup feta cheese crumbles,
  divided
Dash Sriracha-Style Chile Sauce
  (page 162) or store-bought
  (optional)

FAT LOSS: Adding additional fiber can be easily accomplished with more veggies, whole-grain toast, or even avocado on the side (rich in fiber and healthy fats).

1. Preheat the oven to 350°F. Grease a 9 x 13-inch baking pan with butter.

2. In a large skillet over medium heat, warm the olive oil. Add the bell pepper and scallion and cook until both are tender and cooked through, about 8 minutes.

3. Add the spinach and cook until wilted, about 2 minutes. Remove from the heat.

4. In a medium bowl, whisk together the eggs, yogurt, salt, and pepper until blended.

5. Add ¼ cup of feta and the veggies to the egg mixture. Stir to combine.

6. Pour the mixture into the prepared pan. Sprinkle the remaining feta on top.

7. Bake for 25 to 35 minutes, until the eggs have puffed up and the center seems firm.

8. Let cool slightly, then cut. Finish with a dash of hot sauce, if desired.

PER SERVING (1 SQUARE): Calories: 210; Protein: 15g; Total Carbohydrates: 6g; Fiber: 2g; Fat: 14g

MACROS: 26% Protein; 66% Fat; 8% Carbohydrates

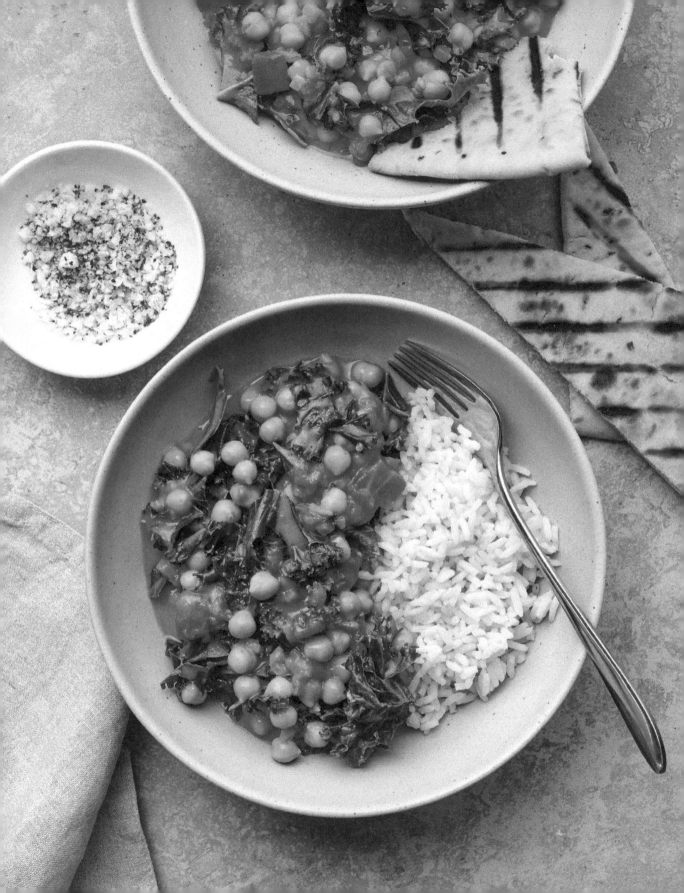

4

PLANT-BASED MEALS

30-Minute Veggie Risotto

PREP TIME: 5 minutes • **COOK TIME:** 35 minutes • **SERVES 4**

While some risotto recipes can be difficult to make and aren't always part of a healthy diet plan, this one allows you to enjoy the creaminess a good risotto provides in a healthier package. You can really make it your own with the vegetables you choose to add—zucchini, cherry tomatoes, asparagus, and bell peppers also work well.

4½ cups unsalted vegetable broth, divided

2 tablespoons olive oil, divided

1 bunch broccolini, trimmed

1 cup chopped mushrooms (such as portobello or shiitake)

Salt

Freshly ground black pepper

1 small shallot, sliced thinly

1 cup Arborio rice

⅓ cup finely grated Parmesan cheese

1. Heat 4 cups of broth in a medium saucepan over medium heat. Once simmering, reduce the heat to low and cover the pot.

2. Heat a large skillet or Dutch oven over medium heat. Add 1 tablespoon of oil, the broccolini, and mushrooms. Cook, stirring frequently, for 3 to 4 minutes. Season with salt and pepper. Remove from the skillet and set aside.

3. In the same skillet over medium heat, add the remaining 1 tablespoon of oil and the shallot. Sauté for 1 to 2 minutes, until the shallot is softened and slightly browned.

4. Add the rice and cook for 1 minute, stirring with a wooden spoon. Add the remaining ½ cup of broth and cook until the rice has absorbed all the liquid, about 2 minutes.

5. Using a large soup ladle, add warmed broth from the covered saucepan to the skillet one ladle at a time. Keep stirring constantly with occasional stops to allow the risotto to come back to a simmer. Keep it at a simmer, not boiling, as boiling will make the rice gummy.

6. Continue this process until the rice is al dente, 15 to 20 minutes.

7. Once the rice is cooked, remove it from the heat and add the Parmesan cheese. Season with salt and pepper to taste.

8. To serve, divide between four bowls. Store leftovers covered in the refrigerator for up to 3 days.

MUSCLE GAIN: To add protein, a great addition is edamame (10 grams of protein per ½ cup). Add shelled edamame in step 2, and you've quickly taken your recipe up a notch.

PER SERVING (⅔ CUP): Calories: 336; Protein: 10g; Total Carbohydrates: 53g; Fiber: 6g; Fat: 10g

MACROS: 10% Protein; 26% Fat; 64% Carbohydrates

Orzo with Broccoli and Pine Nuts

PREP TIME: 15 minutes • **COOK TIME:** 15 minutes • **SERVES 6**

Fiber and protein help us feel full longer. You can add spinach or kale to this dish for added fiber.

Pinch salt
1½ cups orzo
4½ cups broccoli florets
1 garlic clove, peeled
¼ cup pine nuts
½ cup finely grated Parmesan
  cheese
Grated zest and juice of 1 lemon
¼ cup olive oil
¼ cup plain low- or nonfat
  Greek yogurt
Freshly ground black pepper

FAT LOSS: Two cups of raw kale provide a whopping 14 grams of additional fiber; you can add the greens in step 4 and stir until wilted.

1. Fill a large pot with water and a pinch of salt and bring to a boil. Add the orzo and cook until al dente, 8 to 10 minutes. Drain and return the orzo to the pot.

2. Fill a medium pot with 1 inch of water. Add the broccoli florets, cover, and bring to a boil over medium-high heat. Steam for 1 minute. Drain and rinse with cold running water. Drain well.

3. In a blender, combine 1½ cups of cooked broccoli, the garlic, pine nuts, Parmesan, and lemon juice. Pulse to break up the broccoli. Continue pulsing as you drizzle olive oil. Add the yogurt and pulse until smooth.

4. To the pot with the orzo, add the remaining 3 cups of cooked broccoli, lemon zest, and prepared pesto sauce. Stir until incorporated. If the sauce is too thick, you can thin it with water. Season with salt and pepper and serve.

5. You can store any leftovers covered in the refrigerator for up to 3 days.

PER SERVING (ABOUT 1 CUP): Calories: 370; Protein: 13g; Total Carbohydrates: 39g; Fiber: 5g; Fat: 19g

MACROS: 14% Protein; 45% Fat; 41% Carbohydrates

Weeknight Cauliflower Curry

PREP TIME: 10 minutes • **COOK TIME:** 40 minutes • **SERVES 6**

Coconut milk's medium-chain fats can help support weight loss, suppress hunger, support the gut, and improve workout endurance. This dish is great paired with naan or steamed rice.

2 heads cauliflower, cut into florets

2 tablespoons olive oil

1 teaspoon salt

2 tablespoons garam masala, divided

1½ teaspoons ground turmeric, divided

1½ teaspoons ground cinnamon, divided

1½ teaspoons ground coriander, divided

1 teaspoon ground cumin, divided

1½ cups raw cashews

2 tablespoons unsalted butter

1 small onion, chopped

3 garlic cloves, minced

2 cups unsalted vegetable broth

1 cup unsweetened coconut milk

Freshly ground black pepper

MUSCLE GAIN: To increase the total protein in this recipe, firm tofu is a good addition. Add it in step 6, simmering it with the cauliflower for 10 minutes.

1. Preheat the oven to 400°F. On a rimmed baking sheet, toss the cauliflower with the oil, salt, and ½ teaspoon each of garam masala, turmeric, cinnamon, coriander, and cumin. Spread the cauliflower out evenly and roast for 30 minutes, until it's fork-tender.

2. While the cauliflower is roasting, soak the cashews in boiling water for 10 minutes.

3. In a medium pan, melt the butter and sauté the onion and garlic, until fragrant, 1 to 2 minutes. Add the remaining garam masala, turmeric, cinnamon, coriander, and cumin and cook for another 1 to 2 minutes.

4. Drain the cashews. In a blender, combine the cashews, onion mixture, broth, and coconut milk. Blend until smooth. Pour into the same pan. Season with pepper.

5. Add the cauliflower to the pan with the curry sauce and simmer for 10 minutes, then serve. Store leftovers covered in the refrigerator for up to 5 days.

PER SERVING (ABOUT ¾ CUP): Calories: 401; Protein: 11g; Total Carbohydrates: 24g; Fiber: 6g; Fat: 32g

MACROS: 9% Protein; 68% Fat; 23% Carbohydrates

Cauliflower Tacos with Avocado Crema

PREP TIME: 15 minutes • **COOK TIME:** 45 minutes • **SERVES 4**

Street tacos are fun, and you can really play with the spices in this recipe. Try topping these tacos with sliced radishes, pickled jalapeños, and diced onions.

1 head cauliflower, cut into florets

½ small head red cabbage, sliced

¼ cup olive oil

1 teaspoon ground cumin

1 teaspoon salt

1 teaspoon chili powder

½ teaspoon paprika

¼ teaspoon red pepper flakes

1 avocado, peeled, pitted, and roughly chopped

½ cup fresh cilantro

Juice of 1 lime

3 tablespoons plain low- or nonfat Greek yogurt

8 (6-inch) corn tortillas

MUSCLE GAIN: You can increase the total Greek yogurt in this recipe to bump up the protein load and help you meet your daily macro goal.

1. Preheat the oven to 400°F.

2. On a baking sheet, spread the cauliflower and cabbage out in an even layer. Drizzle with the olive oil. Sprinkle with the cumin, salt, chili powder, paprika, and red pepper flakes and mix well. Roast for 45 minutes, until the vegetables are soft and browned, tossing every 15 minutes.

3. For the avocado crema, combine the avocado, cilantro, lime juice, yogurt, and a pinch of salt in a blender and puree until smooth. If the sauce is too thick, add water 1 to 2 teaspoons at a time until it reaches your desired consistency.

4. To serve, divide the roasted vegetables and avocado crema among the tortillas.

5. Store the roasted vegetables in an air-tight container in the refrigerator for up to 3 days. Store the avocado crema in a jar in the refrigerator for up to 1 month.

PER SERVING (2 TACOS): Calories: 372; Protein: 8g; Total Carbohydrates: 40g; Fiber: 9g; Fat: 23g

MACROS: 6% Protein; 54% Fat; 40% Carbohydrates

Sheet-Pan Sweet Potatoes with Crispy Chickpeas

PREP TIME: 10 minutes • **COOK TIME:** 50 minutes • **SERVES 2**

A sheet-pan dinner is always welcome at my house. One that's full of flavor and easy to prep ahead of time—sign me up!

2 medium sweet potatoes, scrubbed and sliced into wedges

3 tablespoons olive oil, divided

2 teaspoons red pepper flakes

Salt

Freshly ground black pepper

1 (15-ounce) can chickpeas, drained and rinsed

1 teaspoon cayenne pepper

1 cup plain low- or nonfat Greek yogurt

Juice of 1 large lime or 2 small limes

Fresh arugula, for serving (optional)

FAT LOSS: This meal also goes nicely on a bed of arugula which keeps the fiber content high, and you can lower the carbs by using less total sweet potato.

1. Preheat the oven to 400°F.

2. In a large bowl, combine the sweet potatoes, 2 tablespoons of oil, and the red pepper flakes. Season with salt and black pepper. Toss until the sweet potato wedges are evenly coated. Place the sweet potatoes on an unlined baking sheet and transfer to the oven. Roast for 25 to 30 minutes, until fork-tender.

3. While the sweet potatoes are roasting, on a second baking sheet, spread the chickpeas out in a single layer. Sprinkle with the cayenne pepper and season with salt and black pepper. Transfer to the oven with the sweet potatoes. Bake until golden brown, about 15 to 20 minutes.

4. For the yogurt sauce, whisk together the yogurt and lime juice in a small bowl. Season to taste with salt and black pepper.

5. Divide the sweet potatoes onto two plates. Top with the crispy chickpeas and drizzle with the yogurt sauce. Serve immediately.

PER SERVING (½ BATCH): Calories: 531; Protein: 14g; Total Carbohydrates: 60g; Fiber: 11g; Fat: 27g

MACROS: 10% Protein; 45% Fat; 45% Carbohydrates

Chickpea and Couscous Salad

PREP TIME: 20 minutes • **COOK TIME:** 15 minutes • **SERVES 6**

Chickpeas are packed with fiber, and they're also an easy and inexpensive way to add protein to any meal or snack. For a bonus, they're a plant-based source of iron, too.

1 (15-ounce) can chickpeas, drained and rinsed
4 tablespoons olive oil, divided
Grated zest and juice of 1 lemon
1 garlic clove, minced
Pinch cayenne pepper
1 cup couscous
1¼ cups water
1 large cucumber, chopped
10 ounces cherry tomatoes, halved
½ red onion, diced finely
1 tablespoon balsamic vinegar
Fresh mint, for garnish (optional)
Feta cheese crumbles, for topping (optional)
Salt
Freshly ground black pepper

1. In a small saucepan over medium heat, combine the chickpeas, 2 tablespoons of olive oil, half of the lemon juice, garlic, and cayenne. Stir until the chickpeas are evenly coated and warmed, about 2 minutes. Set aside.

2. In another saucepan over medium-high heat, add the remaining 2 tablespoons of olive oil and the remaining lemon juice. Once the olive oil and lemon juice become fragrant, 1 to 2 minutes, add the couscous. Toast the couscous for 1 minute, then add the water and stir.

3. Bring the water to a boil, then reduce the heat to low and cover. Let the couscous simmer for 10 minutes, or until all the water has been absorbed.

4. Once the couscous is done, remove it from the heat and fluff it with a fork. Pour the couscous into a bowl and place it in the refrigerator to cool for 15 minutes.

5. While the couscous is cooling, combine the cucumber, tomatoes, onion, lemon zest, vinegar, mint (if using), and feta (if using) in a large salad bowl and toss.

6. Add the cooled couscous and chickpeas to the cooled salad bowl. Toss all the ingredients together until combined. Add salt and pepper to taste and serve.

7. If storing this salad, cover and refrigerate for up to 3 days.

FAT LOSS: If you're at or nearly hitting your carb goal for the day, you can cut back on the total couscous for this meal and focus on the fiber-rich veggies and chickpeas.

PER SERVING (ABOUT 1 CUP): Calories: 263; Protein: 7g; Total Carbohydrates: 36g; Fiber: 5g; Fat: 10g

---

MACROS: 10% Protein; 35% Fat; 55% Carbohydrates

Orzo and Arugula Salad

PREP TIME: 15 minutes • **COOK TIME:** 10 minutes • **SERVES 2**

Fresh, light, and colorful, this can be a great main-course salad, or you can serve it as a side for a dinner party or meal prep. Finish it with "Dress It Up" Salad Dressing or your favorite vinaigrette.

1 cup orzo
2 cups fresh arugula
½ cup chopped fresh mozzarella
¼ cup "Dress It Up" Salad Dressing (page 165) or store-bought
4 oil-packed sun-dried tomatoes, chopped
¼ cup raw walnuts, chopped
Juice of ½ lemon

1. Fill a small saucepan with water and bring to a boil. Add the orzo and cook for 7 to 10 minutes, or until al dente.

2. Put the arugula in a large salad bowl.

3. Once the orzo is done, with a slotted spoon, scoop the hot orzo over the arugula. Add the mozzarella and some of the vinaigrette. Toss to combine. The arugula will begin to wilt and the cheese will melt. Add more vinaigrette to your liking.

4. To serve, top with the sun-dried tomatoes, walnuts, and a squeeze of fresh lemon juice. Enjoy!

5. This meal can be served warm or at room temperature. Store in an airtight container in the refrigerator for up to 2 days.

FAT LOSS: Orzo is one option for this dish, but you can also substitute lentils or quinoa. In just 1 cup of lentils, you'll receive 18 grams of plant-rich protein and 16 grams of fiber.

PER SERVING (½ BATCH): Calories: 444; Protein: 17g; Total Carbohydrates: 67g; Fiber: 5g; Fat: 12g

MACROS: 15% Protein; 25% Fat; 60% Carbohydrates

One-Pot Chickpea Curry

PREP TIME: 10 minutes • **COOK TIME:** 25 minutes • **SERVES 4**

I love this recipe on a cold night paired with pita or rice. Delicious, full of spices, and filling, it makes for a healthy, well-rounded meal with the greens, coconut milk, chickpeas, and tomatoes. This dish comes together in under 30 minutes but tastes like you've been cooking for hours.

2 tablespoons olive oil

3 garlic cloves, minced

1 small onion, minced

1 teaspoon grated fresh ginger

1 (15-ounce) can unsweetened
   coconut milk

½ cup vegetable broth

1 (15-ounce) can diced
   tomatoes

1½ tablespoons tomato paste

2 teaspoons garam masala

¼ teaspoon red pepper flakes

2 (15-ounce) cans chickpeas,
   drained and rinsed

4 cups chopped fresh kale

Salt

Freshly ground black pepper

1. In a large skillet or Dutch oven over medium heat, heat the olive oil. Once the oil is fragrant, add the garlic, onion, and ginger. Sauté for 3 to 5 minutes.

2. Add the coconut milk, broth, tomatoes with their juices, tomato paste, garam masala, and red pepper flakes. Stir to combine. Bring to a boil over medium-high heat.

3. Once boiling, add the chickpeas and reduce the heat to low. Let simmer for 10 minutes.

4. Add the kale and cook for another 2 minutes. Season with salt and black pepper and serve. This saves nicely for leftovers and can be stored in an airtight container in the refrigerator for up to 5 days.

MUSCLE GAIN: Added protein here can come from a variety of sources. One option would be to add firm tofu, cut into chunks and cooked with the chickpeas in step 3. The coconut milk keeps the flavor and richness present in the dish while maintaining the perfect amount of creaminess.

PER SERVING (1 CUP): Calories: 476; Protein: 12g; Total Carbohydrates: 37g; Fiber: 9g; Fat: 33g

MACROS: 9% Protein; 59% Fat; 32% Carbohydrates

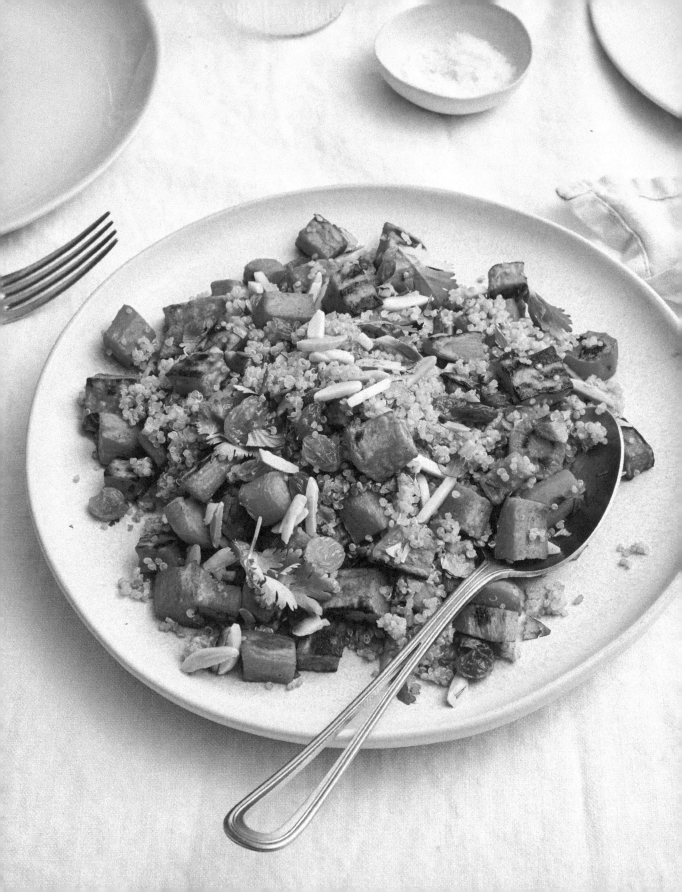

Roasted Vegetable and Quinoa Salad

PREP TIME: 10 minutes • **COOK TIME:** 20 minutes • **SERVES 4**

Roasted root vegetables combined with the warm spices of cumin, cinnamon, and cardamom are perfect for crisp fall nights.

2 sweet potatoes, scrubbed and cut into ½-inch dice

2 carrots, peeled and cut into ½-inch dice

1 tablespoon avocado oil

1 teaspoon garlic powder

1 tablespoon ground cumin

1 teaspoon ground cinnamon

¼ teaspoon salt

¼ teaspoon ground cardamom

2 cups water

1 cup quinoa

¼ cup golden raisins

¼ cup slivered almonds

Grated zest and juice of 1 lemon

MUSCLE GAIN: Add beans, legumes, or tofu to the vegetables for a boost of plant-based protein. You can also pair this meal with Rainbow Hummus (page 160).

1. Preheat the oven to 425°F. Line a baking sheet with parchment paper.

2. In a large bowl, combine the sweet potatoes, carrots, oil, garlic powder, cumin, cinnamon, salt, and cardamom. Toss well to evenly coat the vegetables with the seasoning. Transfer the mixture to the lined baking sheet and spread out in an even layer. Roast for about 20 minutes, or until tender.

3. While the vegetables are roasting, combine the water and quinoa in a medium saucepan. Bring to a boil, reduce the heat, and simmer for about 15 minutes, or until the water is fully absorbed.

4. Combine the cooked quinoa, raisins, and slivered almonds in a bowl. Add the lemon zest and juice and toss. Add the roasted vegetables and toss to combine. Divide among four bowls and serve.

5. This salad stores nicely in an airtight container in the refrigerator for up to 3 days.

PER SERVING (ABOUT ¾ CUP): Calories: 334; Protein: 10g; Total Carbohydrates: 55g; Fiber: 8g; Fat: 10g

MACROS: 10% Protein; 26% Fat; 64% Carbohydrates

Cannellini Bean Ratatouille

PREP TIME: 15 minutes • **COOK TIME:** 20 minutes • **SERVES 4**

Ratatouille is a French stew typically made with summer vegetables, including zucchini, eggplant, tomatoes, onion, and garlic. This dish can be enjoyed hot or cold and is usually served as a side dish. Adding white beans and pine nuts—along with a hearty slice of bread, if you like—makes it a complete meal.

2 tablespoons olive oil

½ yellow onion, chopped

3 garlic cloves, minced

2 tablespoons tomato paste

1 zucchini, cut into 1-inch cubes

1 small yellow squash, cut into 1-inch cubes

1 small eggplant, cut into 1-inch cubes

¼ cup water

½ teaspoon salt

⅛ teaspoon freshly ground black pepper

1 (15-ounce) can fire-roasted diced tomatoes

1 (15-ounce) can cannellini beans, drained and rinsed

¼ cup chopped fresh basil

¼ cup pine nuts, for topping (optional)

¼ cup halved green olives, for topping (optional)

1. Heat the olive oil in a large, deep skillet over medium heat. Add the onion, garlic, and tomato paste and sauté for 2 minutes, or until the onions are translucent. Add the zucchini, yellow squash, and eggplant and sauté for 8 minutes. Halfway through the cooking time, add the water and mix well, scraping the bottom of the skillet.

2. Add the salt, pepper, diced tomatoes with their juices, and beans. Cook for 10 more minutes, then stir in the basil.

3. Divide into four bowls. Top with the pine nuts and olives (if using). Leftovers can be stored in an airtight container in the refrigerator for up to 5 days.

FAT LOSS: The cannellini bean spin to this ratatouille is a way to increase protein and fiber; 1 cup of white beans provides 6 grams of protein and 19 grams of fiber. To bump this up even more, you can add more beans or pair this dish with sautéed spinach for some additional fiber.

PER SERVING (1¼ CUPS): Calories: 302; Protein: 10g; Total Carbohydrates: 35g; Fiber: 12g; Fat: 8g

MACROS: 13% Protein; 30% Fat; 57% Carbohydrates

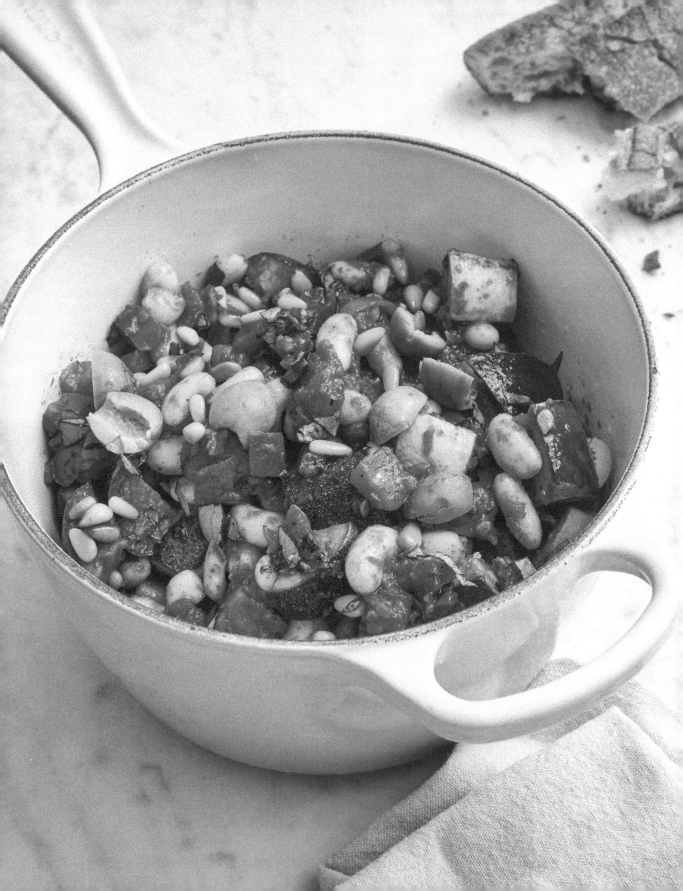

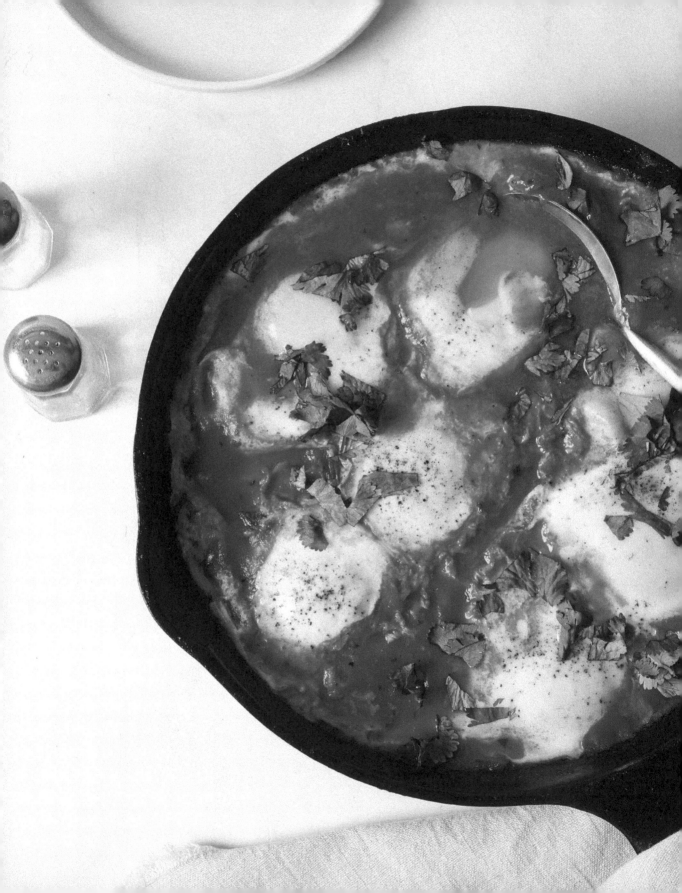

Shakshuka with Spinach

PREP TIME: 10 minutes • **COOK TIME:** 20 minutes • **SERVES 4**

Originating in North Africa and the Middle East, shakshuka is a dish of eggs poached in a sauce made from tomatoes and bell peppers. It is a wonderful, warming meal that comes together quickly. Spinach adds extra nutrients and some bright greens. If it fits into your goals, complete the meal with a slice of crusty whole-grain bread for dipping.

1 tablespoon olive oil
1 small onion, chopped
1 medium red bell pepper, seeded and chopped
3 garlic cloves, minced
2 (15-ounce) cans diced tomatoes
2 cups grated carrots
1½ teaspoons paprika
1 teaspoon ground cumin
½ teaspoon salt
4 cups chopped spinach
8 large eggs
½ cup chopped fresh parsley, for garnish

1. In a large skillet, heat the oil over medium heat. Cook the onion and bell pepper until softened, about 5 minutes, stirring occasionally. Add the garlic and sauté for 30 seconds, until fragrant.

2. Add the tomatoes with their juices and carrots and mix well. Stir in the paprika, cumin, and salt. Simmer for 5 minutes, until slightly thickened.

3. Stir in the spinach. Using a large spoon, make 8 wells in the mixture, evenly spaced throughout the skillet. Crack an egg into each well. Cover and cook for 5 to 8 minutes, until the eggs are cooked to your desired doneness.

4. Garnish with the chopped parsley and serve.

MUSCLE GAIN: For additional protein, you can add an additional egg white on top of each egg in step 3.

PER SERVING (2 EGGS PLUS ABOUT 1 CUP SAUCE): Calories: 268; Protein: 17g; Total Carbohydrates: 21g; Fiber: 8g; Fat: 14g

MACROS: 25% Protein; 48% Fat; 27% Carbohydrates

Halloumi Fajitas

PREP TIME: 10 minutes • **COOK TIME:** 20 minutes • **SERVES 4**

Fajitas are one of the easiest things to put together: You can cook up every-thing in one pan or put it all in the oven. If you're in a time crunch, you can replace the spices with 1 tablespoon of store-bought fajita seasoning mix.

1 green bell pepper, seeded and sliced

1 cup sliced grape tomatoes, divided

½ cup sliced mushrooms

⅓ small white onion, thinly sliced

7 ounces halloumi cheese, cut into strips

1½ teaspoons olive oil

1 teaspoon paprika

½ teaspoon chili powder

½ teaspoon ground cumin

½ teaspoon garlic powder

½ teaspoon onion powder

8 (6-inch) corn tortillas

2 cups shredded lettuce

Lime wedges (optional)

1. Preheat the oven to 450°F. Line a baking sheet with parchment paper.

2. In a large bowl, combine the bell pepper, ½ cup of tomatoes, mushrooms, onion, halloumi, and olive oil. Mix well.

3. In a small bowl, mix the paprika, chili powder, cumin, garlic powder, and onion powder together. Sprinkle the halloumi mixture with the spices. Spread out the mixture on the prepared baking sheet.

4. Bake for 12 to 15 minutes, or until golden brown. Remove the cooked halloumi and continue to cook the vegetables for an additional 5 minutes, or until slightly tender.

5. To assemble, evenly divide the halloumi and vegetables into the tortillas and top with the lettuce. Top with the remaining ½ cup of tomatoes and a squeeze of lime (if using) and serve.

FAT LOSS: To increase this dish's protein and fiber content, consider loading the fajitas with fiber-rich black beans. Whether your goal is muscle gain or fat loss, if you'd like to increase the healthy fats in this recipe, consider adding slices of avocado to your assembled tacos.

PER SERVING (2 TACOS): Calories: 346; Protein: 18g; Total Carbohydrates: 32g; Fiber: 4g; Fat: 17g

MACROS: 20% Protein; 43% Fat; 37% Carbohydrates

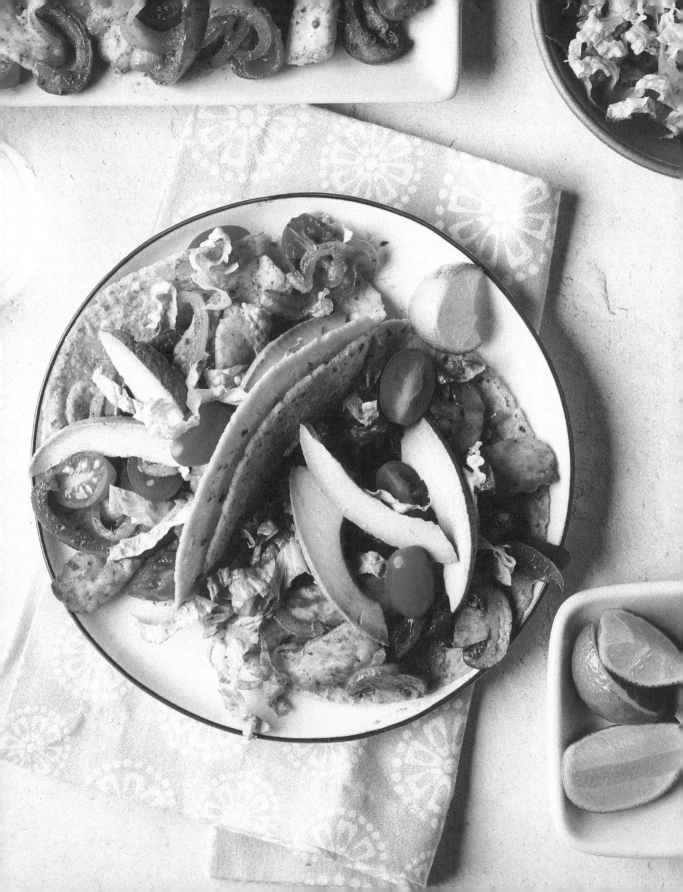

Sweet Potato Chili

PREP TIME: 10 minutes • **COOK TIME:** 45 minutes • **SERVES 4**

A good sweet potato chili gives you all the feels that a meaty chili does but in a much leaner option. The sweet potato is packed with vitamins, minerals, antioxidants, and fiber, while the black beans and quinoa complete the chili for a wholesome, hearty dish.

1 tablespoon olive oil

1 large sweet potato, peeled and diced

1 small onion, diced

2 garlic cloves, minced

2 tablespoons chili powder

1 teaspoon paprika

½ teaspoon ground cumin

¼ teaspoon salt

¼ teaspoon freshly ground black pepper

4 cups vegetable broth

1 (15-ounce) can black beans (or your choice of beans), drained and rinsed

1 (15-ounce) can diced tomatoes

1 cup quinoa

1. Heat the oil in a large skillet or Dutch oven over medium-high heat. Add the sweet potato and onion and cook for about 5 minutes. Add the garlic, chili powder, paprika, cumin, salt, and pepper. Stir to combine.

2. Add the vegetable broth, beans, tomatoes with their juices, and quinoa. Bring to a boil, stirring occasionally.

3. Reduce the heat to low, cover, and simmer for 30 to 35 minutes, until the quinoa is cooked and the potatoes are fork-tender.

4. Remove from the heat and serve. Store leftovers in an airtight container in the refrigerator for up to 5 days.

MUSCLE GAIN: This is really a lean dish to start, and you can easily double up on the beans if you like a bean-forward chili. Adding another 1 cup of black beans will increase the protein by 16 grams; if doing this, you may want to increase the total vegetable broth by an additional cup as well.

PER SERVING (ABOUT 1¼ CUPS): Calories: 340; Protein: 14g; Total Carbohydrates: 57g; Fiber: 14g; Fat: 7g

MACROS: 15% Protein; 19% Fat; 66% Carbohydrates

Quinoa with Roasted Butternut Squash and Feta

PREP TIME: 10 minutes • **COOK TIME:** 30 minutes • **SERVES 4**

Butternut squash has a unique nuttiness that may remind you of a mix between a sweet potato and a crunchy carrot. You can remove the skin if you like, but it is packed with fiber and vitamin A.

½ cup plus 3 tablespoons olive oil, divided

1 teaspoon sugar

1 teaspoon ground cinnamon

½ teaspoon salt

Pinch freshly ground black pepper

2 (1- to 2-pound) butternut squash, seeded and cut into ½-inch slices

1 cup quinoa

2 cups water

2 tablespoons apple cider vinegar

2 garlic cloves, minced

4 cups fresh arugula

¾ cup feta cheese crumbles

FAT LOSS: To increase fiber and protein, you can increase the total amount of quinoa you prepare and cut back on the feta on top.

1. Preheat the oven to 450°F.

2. In a large bowl, mix 3 tablespoons of olive oil with the sugar, cinnamon, salt, and pepper. Add the squash to the bowl and coat well. Spread the squash out on a rimmed baking sheet.

3. Roast the squash for 10 to 15 minutes, until slightly golden. Turn each slice and continue to roast for another 10 to 15 minutes.

4. While the squash is roasting, combine the quinoa and water in a medium pot. Bring to a boil over medium-high heat, then cover, reduce the heat, and simmer for 10 minutes. Set aside, covered.

5. In a large bowl, combine the vinegar and garlic. Whisk in the remaining ½ cup of olive oil. Season with salt and pepper.

6. Divide the quinoa between four plates. Top with the arugula, squash mixture, and feta, then serve.

PER SERVING (½ CUP QUINOA, 1 CUP ARUGULA, AND ABOUT ¾ CUP SQUASH): Calories: 576; Protein: 12g; Total Carbohydrates: 47g; Fiber: 6g; Fat: 39g

MACROS: 8% Protein; 60% Fat; 32% Carbohydrates

Chickpea and Pear Kale Salad

PREP TIME: 5 minutes • **SERVES 2**

With a bit of spice, crunch, and sweetness, this salad is perfect for when you need something quick or as a side to your main meal. With Roasted Chickpeas and "Dress It Up" Salad Dressing ready to go in your pantry, you can whip this salad up in under 5 minutes.

1 bunch curly kale, stemmed and torn (about 2 cups)

1½ cups Roasted Chickpeas (page 137)

2 firm pears, cored and sliced

2 ounces goat cheese, crumbled (optional)

¼ cup "Dress It Up" Salad Dressing (page 165) or store-bought

1. Put the kale in a large salad bowl. Top with the chickpeas, pears, and goat cheese (if using).

2. Add the salad dressing, toss, and enjoy!

3. If meal prepping, hold off on dressing the salad. Store the salad in an airtight container in the refrigerator for up to 3 days, then add the dressing just before you're ready to eat.

MUSCLE GAIN: If you're looking to add vegetarian protein to this salad, you can top it with some slivered almonds—¼ cup will provide an additional 7 grams of protein.

PER SERVING (½ BATCH): Calories: 398; Protein: 17g; Total Carbohydrates: 60g; Fiber: 13g; Fat: 13g

MACROS: 11% Protein; 22% Fat; 67% Carbohydrates

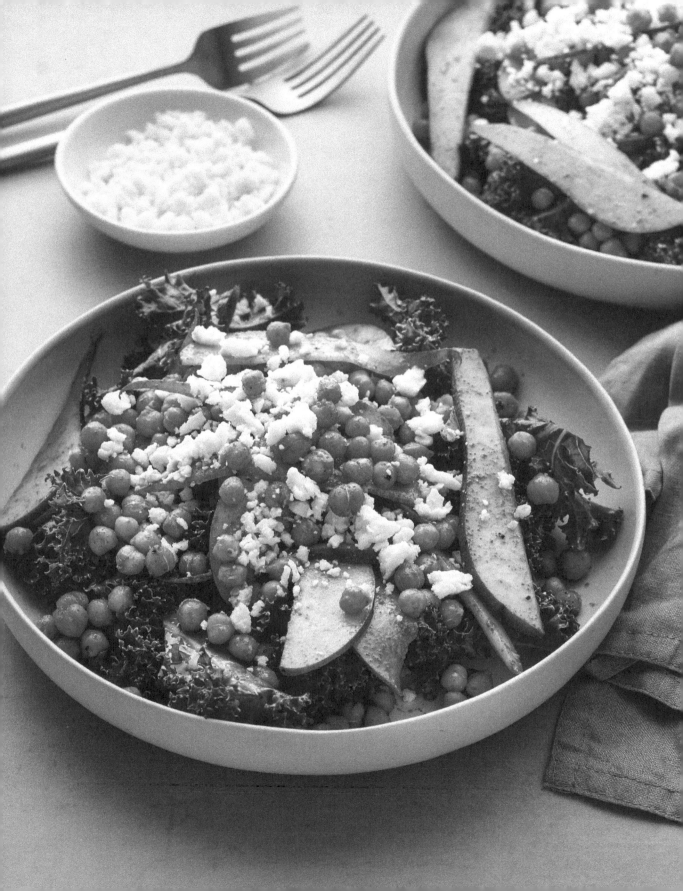

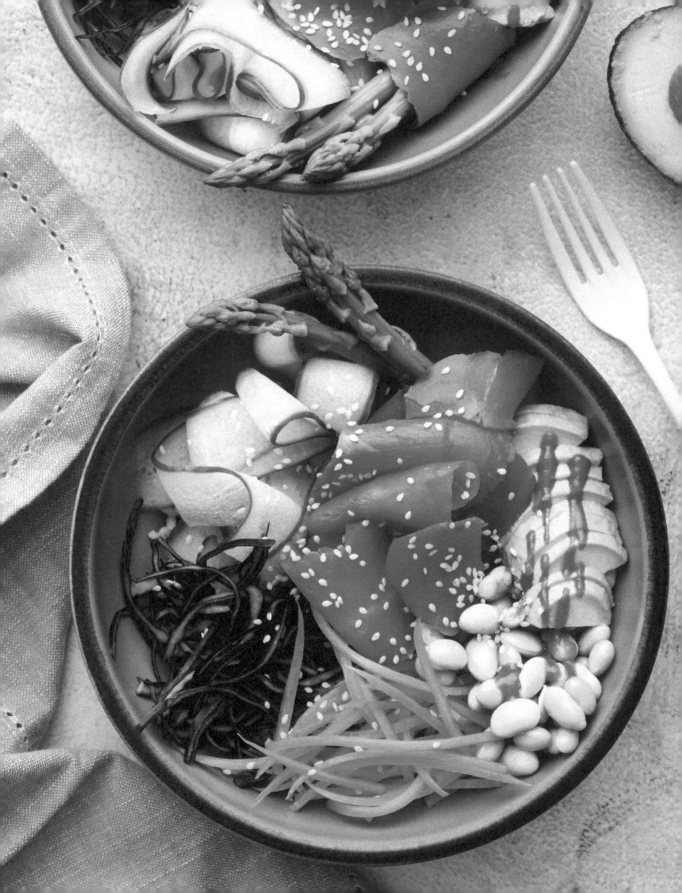

5

SEAFOOD AND POULTRY MEALS

Easy Tuna Niçoise Salad

PREP TIME: 10 minutes • **COOK TIME:** 30 minutes • **SERVES 4**

Tuna is a nutrition powerhouse, rich in vitamins, minerals, omega-3 fats, and protein. Because tuna is a predator fish in the ocean, it will contain mercury, which is why it's important to limit tuna consumption to a few times a week. Yellowfin and albacore tend to have higher mercury content, whereas skipjack tends to be a bit lower.

Nonstick cooking spray
2 cups baby red potatoes, halved or quartered
2 tablespoons olive oil, divided
¼ teaspoon garlic powder
Salt
12 ounces or 3 cups fresh green beans, trimmed
6 cups arugula
1½ cups cherry tomatoes, halved
4 Perfect Hard-Boiled Eggs (page 156), peeled and halved
¾ cup pitted Kalamata olives
2 (5-ounce) cans water-packed tuna, drained and flaked
½ cup "Dress It Up" Salad Dressing (page 165) or store-bought
Freshly ground black pepper

1. Preheat the oven to 400°F. Prep a rimmed baking sheet with nonstick spray.

2. In a large bowl, combine the potatoes, 1 tablespoon of oil, the garlic powder, and a pinch of salt. Mix to coat the potatoes with the seasoning.

3. Spread the potatoes out on the prepared baking sheet and roast for 15 minutes.

4. While the potatoes are roasting, put the green beans in the same bowl that you mixed the potatoes in. Add the remaining 1 tablespoon of oil and another pinch of salt. Toss to coat.

5. Once the potatoes have roasted for 15 minutes, remove the baking sheet from the oven and add the green beans. Try to spread everything out in a single layer.

6. Return the baking sheet to the oven and roast for another 10 to 15 minutes, or until the potatoes are crispy on the outside, but soft in the middle.

7. Remove from the oven and set aside to cool.

8. To assemble the salads, divide the arugula among four plates. Top each plate with equal amounts of tomatoes, egg halves, olives, tuna, and roasted vegetables. Drizzle with the dressing and serve.

9. If meal prepping, hold off on dressing the salad. Store the salad in an airtight container in the refrigerator for up to 3 days, then add the dressing when you're ready to eat.

FAT LOSS: If you're hitting your carb target for the day, you can reduce or omit the red potatoes in this salad.

PER SERVING (¼ BATCH WITH 2 TABLESPOONS DRESSING): Calories: 398; Protein: 27g; Total Carbohydrates: 27g; Fiber: 6g; Fat: 22g

---

MACROS: 26% Protein; 48% Fat; 26% Carbohydrates

Tuna Power Wraps

PREP TIME: 10 minutes • **SERVES 4**

A go-to for lunch, these wraps are packed with protein from the tuna, eggs, and Greek yogurt. The yogurt also adds an incredible creaminess that ties everything together.

2 (5-ounce) cans water-packed tuna, drained

4 Perfect Hard-Boiled Eggs (page 156), peeled and chopped

4 celery stalks, finely chopped

½ cup plain low- or nonfat Greek yogurt

½ cup chopped red onion

2 teaspoons whole-grain mustard

Salt

Freshly ground black pepper

4 large whole-grain tortillas

1 cup alfalfa sprouts

2 small ripe tomatoes, sliced

1. In a large bowl, break apart the tuna. Mix in the eggs, celery, yogurt, onion, and mustard. Season with salt and pepper.

2. Split the mixture between the tortillas and top with the alfalfa sprouts and tomatoes. Fold the sides in, roll the tortillas up, and serve.

FAT LOSS: You can make this recipe more fiber-forward by replacing the alfalfa sprouts with chopped romaine or spinach. When buying whole-grain tortillas, choose the ones with the highest amount of fiber listed per serving.

PER SERVING (1 WRAP): Calories: 289; Protein: 24g; Total Carbohydrates: 25g; Fiber: 5g; Fat: 9g

MACROS: 33% Protein; 33% Fat; 34% Carbohydrates

Blackened Fish Tacos

PREP TIME: 5 minutes • **COOK TIME:** 10 minutes • **SERVES 4**

*Everyone loves a good fish taco. These are quick, easy, and full of flavor.
Pair with a salad and you have yourself a complete meal. Garnish them with
your favorite taco toppings, such as avocado, salsa, crema, lime wedges,
and shredded cabbage.*

1 tablespoon paprika

1 teaspoon salt

1 teaspoon freshly ground black
pepper

½ teaspoon cayenne pepper

½ teaspoon garlic powder

2 tablespoons olive oil

1½ pounds flaky white fish
fillets, such as mahi-mahi
or halibut

8 whole-grain tortillas

1. Heat a grill or grill pan to high heat.

2. In a small bowl, combine the paprika, salt,
black pepper, cayenne, and garlic powder,
then season the fish all over with the spice
mixture. Rub the olive oil into the fish.

3. Grill the fish for 4 minutes per side. If the
fish is thick, it may need 1 to 2 additional
minutes. Once both sides are cooked,
remove the fish from the grill and let cool
for 2 minutes, then flake the fish with a fork.

4. To assemble the tacos, add the flaked fish
to each tortilla.

MUSCLE GAIN: To bump up the protein, increase the
amount of fish (with additional spices) that you add to
each taco. This is a great post-workout dish and perfect
for summer nights.

PER SERVING (2 TACOS): Calories: 475; Protein: 40g; Total
Carbohydrates: 39g; Fiber: 9g; Fat: 17g

MACROS: 35% Protein; 32% Fat; 33% Carbohydrates

Sheet-Pan Fish with Broccoli

PREP TIME: 30 minutes • **COOK TIME:** 30 minutes • **SERVES 4**

The fish in this dish is light and the veggies round out the meal. The broccoli works well for roasting, but you could also sub in zucchini, carrots, mushrooms, green beans—you name it!

½ cup low-sodium soy sauce
1 tablespoon brown sugar
1 teaspoon sesame oil
1½ pounds fish fillets, such as
  sea bass or cod
1 head broccoli, cut into florets
1 tablespoon olive oil
Salt
Freshly ground black pepper

FAT LOSS: To increase the total fiber, add your favorite whole grain on the side.

1. Preheat the oven to 400°F.

2. In a shallow bowl, combine the soy sauce, brown sugar, and sesame oil. Add the fish and allow to sit at room temperature for 30 minutes or covered in the refrigerator overnight.

3. On a rimmed baking sheet, spread the broccoli out in an even layer. Toss with the oil and season with salt and pepper. Roast for 5 to 7 minutes.

4. Remove the baking sheet from the oven and move the broccoli to one side. Add the fish fillets to the empty side. Return to the oven and roast for 12 to 15 minutes. You can brush some marinade onto the fish halfway through if the fish is starting to look a bit dry.

5. Remove from the oven, let rest for 3 to 5 minutes, then serve.

PER SERVING (6 OZ FISH AND ½ CUP BROCCOLI):
Calories: 234; Protein: 35g; Total Carbohydrates: 12g;
Fiber: 5g; Fat: 5g

MACROS: 61% Protein; 21% Fat; 18% Carbohydrates

Oven-Roasted Fish with Burst Tomatoes

PREP TIME: 5 minutes • **COOK TIME:** 20 minutes • **SERVES 4**

"Burst tomatoes" recipes have really hit the cooking scene as of late, and for good reason. This dish is super simple, full of flavor, and looks incredible. Add a perfect fillet of fish and you have yourself a lean, healthy one-pan meal.

1 pint cherry tomatoes, halved
Salt
Freshly ground black pepper
6 tablespoons unsalted butter, melted
2 garlic cloves, minced
½ teaspoon paprika
½ teaspoon onion powder
½ teaspoon grated fresh ginger
1½ pounds fish fillets, such as cod, salmon, or halibut
1 scallion, thinly sliced
Juice of 1 lemon

FAT LOSS: For additional fiber, you can pair this recipe with a green salad (such as arugula, spinach, romaine, or butter lettuce) topped with "Dress It Up" Salad Dressing (page 165).

1. Preheat the oven to 450°F.

2. Place the tomatoes on a rimmed baking sheet. Sprinkle with salt and pepper and roast for 10 minutes.

3. In a small bowl, combine the butter, garlic, paprika, onion powder, ginger, and a pinch of salt.

4. Remove the pan from the oven. Nestle the fish among the tomatoes. Pour the spice mixture over everything, tossing the tomatoes to cover them. Sprinkle the scallions over the top.

5. Roast for 5 to 10 minutes, until the fish is flaky and cooked through. Dress with lemon juice and serve. Leftovers can be stored in an airtight container in the refrigerator for up to 3 days.

PER SERVING (6 OZ FISH AND ½ CUP TOMATOES):
Calories: 422; Protein: 35g; Total Carbohydrates: 6g; Fiber: 2g; Fat: 28g

MACROS: 35% Protein; 60% Fat; 5% Carbohydrates

Shrimp Scampi with Whole-Grain Pasta

PREP TIME: 10 minutes • **COOK TIME:** 10 minutes • **SERVES 4**

Shrimp scampi is a classic dish that's typically loaded with saturated fat from the butter, but this version uses olive oil and some of the starchy water left over from cooking the pasta to create a flavorful sauce that clings to the noodles. Serve this dish with a side of roasted green beans, asparagus, or broccoli for a complete meal.

6 ounces whole-grain linguine or spaghetti

2 tablespoons olive oil

3 garlic cloves, minced

1 cup diced zucchini

12 ounces shrimp, peeled and deveined

Grated zest and juice of 1 lemon

½ cup shredded Parmesan cheese

½ cup chopped fresh parsley

FAT LOSS: To increase the total fiber content, you can keep the pasta amount the same or cut it down to 4 ounces and add 3 to 4 cups of shredded or spiralized zucchini to the skillet in step 3, along with the pasta, then stir until heated through.

1. Bring a large pot of water to a boil over high heat. Cook the pasta according to the package directions, until al dente. Drain, reserving 1 cup of pasta water.

2. Meanwhile, in a large skillet over medium heat, heat the oil. Add the garlic and cook for 30 seconds, until fragrant. Add the zucchini and cook for 3 to 4 minutes, until soft. Add the shrimp and sauté for 4 to 6 minutes, until pink and cooked through. Turn off the heat and sprinkle the mixture with the lemon zest and juice. Stir to combine.

3. Add the pasta to the skillet and stir to mix, adding about ½ cup of the reserved pasta water to create a loose sauce. Add the remaining water, as needed, to thin the sauce and coat the pasta. Sprinkle with the Parmesan and parsley and serve. Leftovers can be stored in an airtight container in the refrigerator for up to 3 days.

PER SERVING (½ CUP PASTA AND 3 SHRIMP): Calories: 346; Protein: 28g; Total Carbohydrates: 38g; Fiber: 5g; Fat: 11g

MACROS: 31% Protein; 29% Fat; 40% Carbohydrates

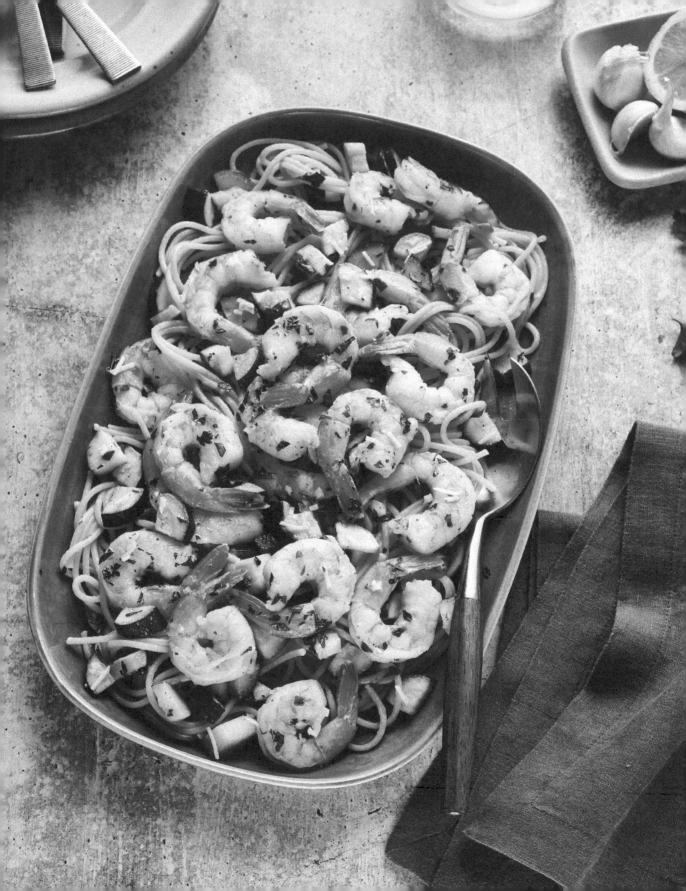

Macro-Friendly Fish 'n' Chips

PREP TIME: 10 minutes • **COOK TIME:** 25 minutes • **SERVES 4**

This one took a while to perfect. Good, authentic fish 'n' chips is hard to beat, and this recipe gives it a healthful spin. Enjoy in moderation, and when it fits your macros.

Nonstick cooking spray
2 tablespoons olive oil, divided
½ teaspoon onion powder, divided
½ teaspoon garlic salt, divided
½ teaspoon freshly ground black pepper, divided
2 large sweet potatoes, scrubbed and cut into ½-inch wedges
½ cup whole-wheat panko breadcrumbs
1 pound (1-inch-thick) cod fillets, cut into strips
Lemon wedges, for serving
Malt vinegar, for serving

FAT LOSS: To add fiber while keeping the fish 'n' chips the stars of the dish, pair this with a salad or steamed veggies.

1. Preheat oven to 425°F. Lightly coat a rimmed baking sheet with nonstick spray.

2. In a large bowl, combine 1 tablespoon of olive oil and ¼ teaspoon each of onion powder, garlic salt, and pepper. Add the sweet potato wedges and toss to coat. Place in a single layer on half of the prepared baking sheet. Bake for 15 minutes.

3. In a small bowl, combine the breadcrumbs, remaining 1 tablespoon of olive oil, and remaining ¼ teaspoon each of onion powder, garlic salt, and pepper. Toss to combine.

4. Remove the baking sheet from the oven. Flip the potato wedges and place the fish on the other half of the baking sheet. Sprinkle the breadcrumb mixture over the fish and return the pan to the oven.

5. Bake for 10 more minutes, or until the potatoes are tender and the fish flakes easily. Serve with lemon wedges or malt vinegar.

PER SERVING (½ SWEET POTATO AND 4 OZ FISH):
Calories: 242; Protein: 22g; Total Carbohydrates: 19g; Fiber: 3g; Fat: 9g

MACROS: 39% Protein; 29% Fat; 32% Carbohydrates

Salmon Poke Bowls

PREP TIME: 10 minutes • **COOK TIME:** 5 minutes • **SERVES 4**

I like to pair this dish with steamed brown rice or even cauliflower rice. When using brown rice, it's good to prep the rice ahead of time as it can be time-consuming to make. That way, these poke bowls can be put together in less than 10 minutes.

8 asparagus spears

2 cups cooked brown rice

1 pound smoked salmon

1 large cucumber, thinly sliced

1 cup edamame, shelled

1 avocado, peeled, pitted, and sliced

2 large carrots, shredded or thinly sliced

½ head purple cabbage, shredded

Sesame seeds (optional)

Sriracha-Style Chile Sauce (page 162) or store-bought (optional)

1. Fill a medium saucepan with 1 to 2 inches of water and bring to a boil over medium heat. Add the asparagus, cover, and steam for about 3 minutes, until bright green. Remove from the heat and rinse under cold water to stop the cooking process. Set aside.

2. Place ½ cup of brown rice in each bowl first. Top with the salmon, cucumber, edamame, avocado, carrots, and cabbage.

3. If desired, sprinkle with sesame seeds for an added crunch, and drizzle with some chile sauce for spice.

MUSCLE GAIN: Make sure to include the brown rice or another whole-grain carb. When aiming for muscle gain, consuming adequate amounts of carbs is critical to make sure you have the energy to fuel your workouts.

PER SERVING (4 OZ SALMON AND ¼ VEGETABLES):
Calories: 315; Protein: 28g; Total Carbohydrates: 21g; Fiber: 9g; Fat: 15g

MACROS: 36% Protein; 40% Fat; 24% Carbohydrates

Crunchy Kale and Salmon Salad

PREP TIME: 5 minutes • **COOK TIME:** 5 minutes • **SERVES 4**

A delicious salmon salad completes any lunch or dinner. I love this recipe, with the tangy dressing, pan-seared salmon, and creamy avocado. Adding seeds, nuts, or quinoa is a great way to add crunch and a bit of fiber.

1 pound salmon, cut into 4-ounce fillets

Salt

Freshly ground black pepper

¼ cup plus 1 tablespoon olive oil, divided

1 garlic clove, minced

⅓ cup finely grated Parmesan cheese

Grated zest and juice of 1 lemon

¼ teaspoon red pepper flakes

3 bunches kale, stemmed and chopped

1 avocado, peeled, pitted, and sliced

1. Sprinkle the salmon fillets with salt and black pepper.

2. Heat 1 tablespoon of olive oil in a medium skillet over high heat. Add the fish and cook for 2 to 3 minutes, until it forms a golden crust. Flip the salmon and cook for another 1 to 2 minutes. Remove and set aside.

3. In a small bowl, combine the garlic, cheese, remaining ¼ cup of olive oil, lemon zest and juice, red pepper flakes, and a pinch of salt and black pepper. Mix to combine.

4. Put the kale in a large salad bowl, add the oil mixture, and toss to combine. Top with the salmon and avocado and serve. Dressed salad can be stored in an air-tight container in the refrigerator for up to 3 days.

MUSCLE GAIN: Sprinkling the salad with pumpkin seeds adds another layer of texture, as well as protein—9 additional grams per ¼ cup.

PER SERVING (¼ BATCH WITH 4 OZ SALMON): Calories: 438; Protein: 29g; Total Carbohydrates: 12g; Fiber: 4g; Fat: 32g

MACROS: 26% Protein; 64% Fat; 10% Carbohydrates

Turkey-Stuffed Peppers

PREP TIME: 10 minutes • **COOK TIME:** 30 minutes • **SERVES 2**

These stuffed peppers will fit into your busy week perfectly. They're easy to make, great for meal prep, and loaded with flavor, color, and protein. You can pair them with a vibrant salad or a side of black beans for added fiber, and voilà, you have a complete meal in minutes.

4 green bell peppers (or your choice of color)
1 tablespoon olive oil
½ onion, finely chopped
1 teaspoon minced garlic
1 pound ground turkey
1 teaspoon paprika
½ teaspoon chili powder
½ teaspoon freshly ground black pepper
Pinch cayenne pepper
1 cup spinach

FAT LOSS: You can cut the total meat in half or focus on non-meat, high-fiber choices, such as lentils or beans. If meal prepping, follow the recipe as described up until the bake step. Store the prepped peppers in your freezer for up to 3 months.

1. Preheat the oven to 425°F.

2. Cut the tops off the peppers and remove the seeds and ribs. Chop the tops (discard the stems). Set aside.

3. Heat the oil in a medium sauté pan over medium heat. Add the onion and garlic and sauté until fragrant, about 2 minutes.

4. Add the turkey, paprika, chili powder, black pepper, and cayenne and cook, stirring frequently, until the turkey is fully browned, about 8 minutes. Add the spinach and chopped pepper tops. Mix to combine and wilt the spinach.

5. Once the spinach has wilted, turn off the heat. With a spoon, stuff each pepper shell with the meat mixture. Place the stuffed peppers in a roasting pan and bake until tender, about 20 minutes.

6. Serve hot and enjoy!

PER SERVING (2 PEPPERS): Calories: 465; Protein: 48g; Total Carbohydrates: 16g; Fiber: 6g; Fat: 25g

MACROS: 40% Protein; 48% Fat; 12% Carbohydrates

Turkey Sweet Potato Skins

PREP TIME: 10 minutes • **COOK TIME:** 1 hour 30 minutes • **SERVES 4**

Potato skins make for a great meal-prep option or tailgate snack. These turkey-filled sweet potato skins have the perfect amount of spice without all the added saturated fat you may find in a classic potato skin recipe.

4 medium sweet potatoes, well scrubbed

3 tablespoons olive oil, divided

12 ounces ground turkey or chicken

2 garlic cloves, minced

2 teaspoons chili powder

1 teaspoon smoked paprika

1 teaspoon ground cumin

½ teaspoon salt

3 cups spinach

Juice of 1 lime

Freshly ground black pepper

1. Preheat the oven to 425°F.

2. Prick the sweet potatoes all over with a fork. Place them directly on the oven rack and bake for 50 to 60 minutes, until fork-tender.

3. While the potatoes are baking, in a large skillet over medium heat, heat 2 tablespoons of oil. Add the turkey and cook until completely browned, about 8 minutes. Add the garlic, chili powder, paprika, cumin, and salt. Stir and cook for another 5 minutes, until fragrant.

4. Add the spinach and cook until wilted, about 2 to 3 minutes. Remove the skillet from the heat and stir in the lime juice.

5. Remove the sweet potatoes from the oven. Cut them in half lengthwise. (Be careful, as they will be hot.) Let them cool for up to 5 minutes, then scoop out some flesh but leave enough to ensure the potatoes do not collapse.

6. Place the skins in a roasting pan, flesh-side up. Brush the potatoes with the remaining 1 tablespoon of olive oil and season with salt and pepper. Bake for 5 to 10 minutes, or until crisp.

7. Remove the skins from the oven and stuff them with the turkey mixture. Return to the oven for another 10 minutes, until the skins are nice and crispy.

MUSCLE GAIN: To increase the protein content for these potato skins, you have a few different options. You could bump up the total meat to 1 pound; you could add 1 cup of black beans when you add the garlic and spices in step 3; or you could top the skins with plain low- or nonfat Greek yogurt or shredded Cheddar cheese.

PER SERVING (2 SWEET POTATO HALVES): Calories: 345; Protein: 20g; Total Carbohydrates: 30g; Fiber: 5g; Fat: 17g

MACROS: 22% Protein; 44% Fat; 34% Carbohydrates

Turkey and Veggie Burgers with Sweet Potatoes

PREP TIME: 15 minutes • **COOK TIME:** 25 minutes • **SERVES 8**

The mushrooms, carrots, and zucchini make this turkey burger unique. Top with avocado, lettuce, red onion, pickles, Rainbow Hummus (page 160), or Macro-Friendly Ketchup (page 163).

2 sweet potatoes, scrubbed and cut into ½-inch wedges

1 tablespoon olive oil

¼ teaspoon salt

1 pound ground turkey

Freshly ground black pepper

½ cup finely chopped mushrooms

¾ cup grated carrots

¾ cup grated zucchini

3 garlic cloves, minced

½ onion, minced

8 whole-wheat hamburger buns

MUSCLE GAIN: To add more protein, you can always fancy these burgers up with a fried egg on top.

1. Preheat the oven to 425°F. Line a rimmed baking sheet with parchment paper.

2. In a medium bowl, toss together the sweet potatoes, olive oil, and salt. Stir to combine. Place the sweet potatoes on the baking sheet and roast for 25 minutes, flipping halfway through.

3. Meanwhile, in a large bowl, mix the turkey, a pinch each of salt and pepper, mushrooms, carrots, zucchini, garlic, and onion. Shape into 8 patties.

4. Warm a grill or grill pan to medium heat. Brush the grates with olive oil to prevent sticking and cook the patties for 6 minutes on each side, or until they reach an internal temperature of 165°F.

5. Serve the burgers on the buns with the sweet potato wedges on the side. You can store leftover cooked patties in an airtight container in the refrigerator for up to 5 days, or freeze uncooked patties for up to 6 months.

PER SERVING (1 BURGER AND ½ SWEET POTATO): Calories: 254; Protein: 16g; Total Carbohydrates: 31g; Fiber: 5g; Fat: 8g

MACROS: 24% Protein; 28% Fat; 48% Carbohydrates

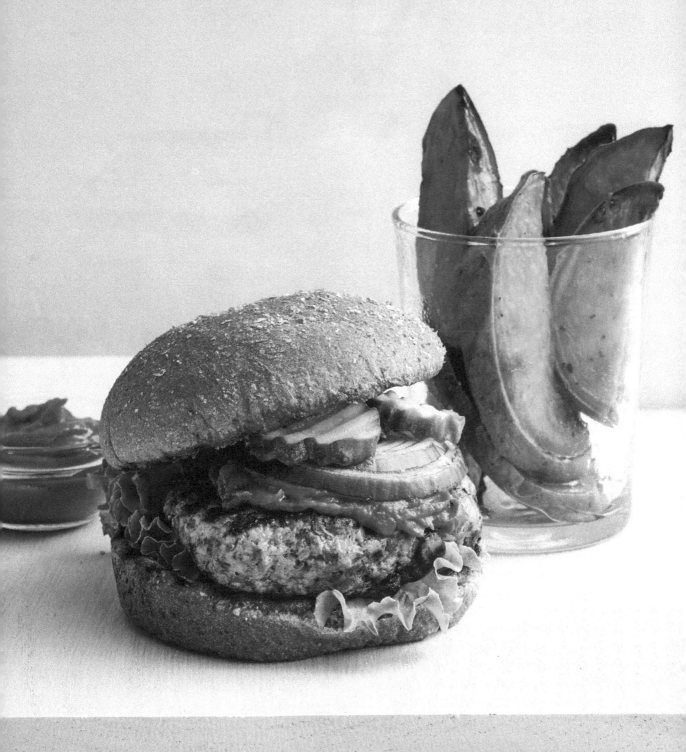

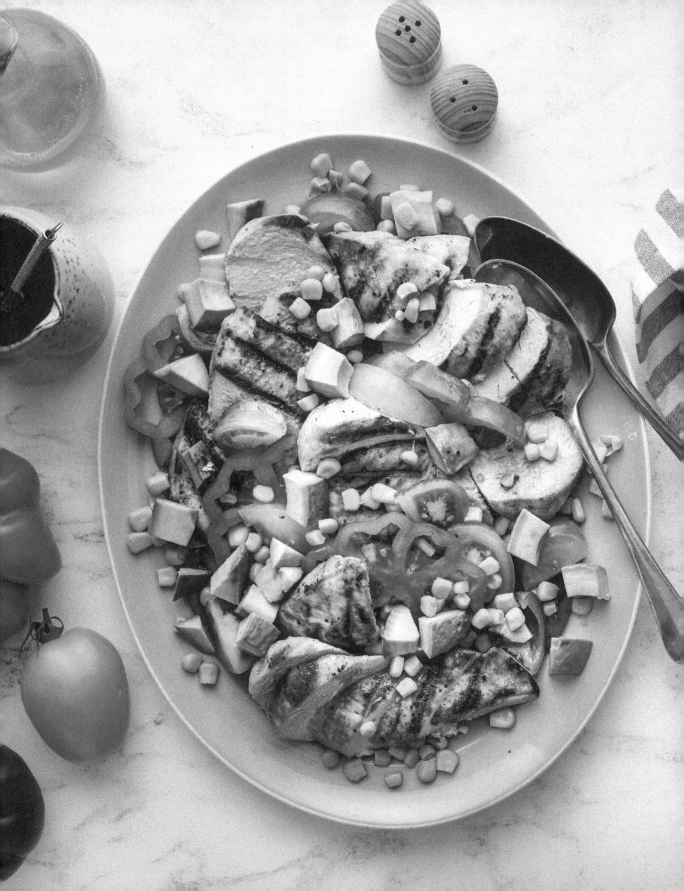

Grilled Chicken with Avocado and Tomato Salad

PREP TIME: 45 minutes • **COOK TIME:** 15 minutes • **SERVES 4**

This is a clean, fresh, healthy meal. I love it on summer nights when heir-loom tomatoes are at their peak ripeness. You can grill or boil fresh corn on the cob, or if you're in a time crunch, frozen corn kernels work great as well.

¼ cup olive oil

Juice of 1 lime

½ teaspoon salt

½ teaspoon freshly ground black pepper

4 boneless, skinless chicken breasts

2 avocados, peeled, pitted, and diced

3 or 4 heirloom tomatoes, sliced or cut into wedges

1 cup fresh or frozen corn kernels

¼ cup "Dress It Up" Salad Dressing (page 165) or store-bought (optional)

1. In a shallow dish, combine the olive oil, lime juice, salt, and pepper. Stir to combine. Add the chicken and turn to coat well. Marinate for 30 to 45 minutes at room temperature.

2. Heat a grill or grill pan to high heat. Remove the chicken from the marinade, discarding the marinade. Cook the chicken for about 8 minutes on each side, until no longer pink in the middle with an internal temperature of 165°F.

3. Transfer the chicken to a platter and cut into thick slices. Top with the avocado, tomatoes, and corn. Sprinkle with salt and pepper and drizzle with dressing (if using).

MUSCLE GAIN: This is a high-protein, lower-carb meal. To increase the carb load, you can pair it with quinoa, lentils, or even a side of pasta.

PER SERVING (¼ VEGETABLES WITH 1 CHICKEN BREAST): Calories: 437; Protein: 30g; Total Carbohydrates: 22g; Fiber: 9g; Fat: 27g

MACROS: 28% Protein; 53% Fat; 19% Carbohydrates

Chicken-Vegetable Udon Noodle Stir-Fry

PREP TIME: 15 minutes • **COOK TIME:** 20 minutes • **SERVES 6**

Udon noodles are a thick, chewy, whole-wheat Japanese pasta. Customize this with edamame, bean sprouts, sesame seeds, and cilantro for a flavor boost.

1 (8-ounce) package whole-grain udon noodles

1 tablespoon olive oil

3 garlic cloves, minced

1 small bunch scallions, sliced

1 baby bok choy, chopped

1 carrot, julienned

6 ounces shiitake mushrooms, sliced

1 tablespoon sesame oil

1 pound boneless, skinless chicken breast, cut into ½-inch strips

¼ cup chicken broth

2 tablespoons low-sodium soy sauce

1 tablespoon rice vinegar

¼ cup peanuts

MUSCLE GAIN: The peanuts and chicken are great protein sources in this recipe. To heighten the peanut flavor and add 14 grams of protein, you can add 2 tablespoons of peanut butter in step 4.

1. Put the noodles in a medium saucepan and add enough water to cover them. Bring to a boil and cook for 11 minutes. Drain the noodles and set aside.

2. While the noodles are cooking, heat the olive oil in a wok or deep skillet. Add the garlic and scallions and sauté for 3 minutes. Add the bok choy, carrot, and mushrooms and sauté for another 5 minutes. Remove the vegetables and set aside.

3. In the same wok over medium heat, heat the sesame oil and add the chicken. Cook for 5 minutes.

4. Return the vegetables to the wok and sauté for 2 minutes. Add the cooked udon noodles, broth, soy sauce, rice vinegar, and peanuts. Mix well and sauté for an additional 5 minutes. This dish can be stored in an airtight container in the refrigerator for up to 3 days.

PER SERVING (4 OZ CHICKEN WITH 2 OZ NOODLES AND ⅙ VEGETABLES): Calories: 327; Protein: 23g; Total Carbohydrates: 34g; Fiber: 3g; Fat: 10g

MACROS: 32% Protein; 28% Fat; 40% Carbohydrates

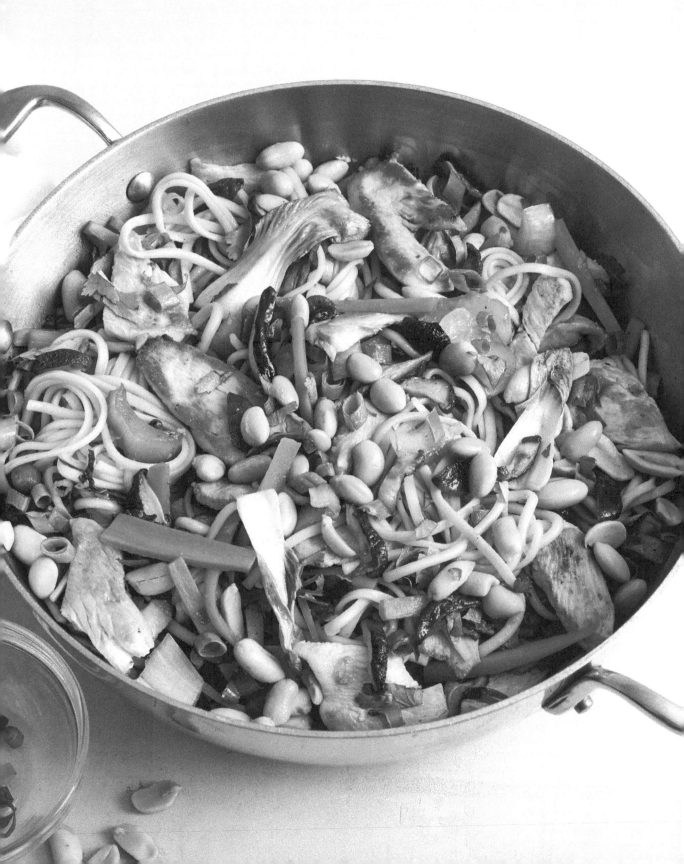

Spiced Chicken Meatballs

PREP TIME: 10 minutes • **COOK TIME:** 10 minutes • **SERVES 4**

This recipe provides a lean, protein-rich meatball with delicious spices and creamy yogurt. I like to cover my plate with arugula, then top with meatballs and yogurt, with a side of Rainbow Hummus (page 160) and Homemade Pita Chips (page 155).

1½ cups plain low- or nonfat
   Greek yogurt, divided
3 garlic cloves, minced, divided
Juice from 1 lemon
Salt
Freshly ground black pepper
1 pound ground chicken
½ cup whole-wheat panko
   breadcrumbs
1 large egg, beaten
2 tablespoons olive oil, divided
1 tablespoon dried parsley
1 teaspoon paprika
½ teaspoon ground cumin
½ teaspoon grated fresh ginger
½ teaspoon ground cinnamon
Fresh arugula, for serving

1. Combine 1 cup of yogurt, one-third of the garlic, the lemon juice, and a pinch each of salt and pepper in a small bowl. Mix well. Place in the refrigerator to chill until ready to serve.

2. In a large bowl, combine the remaining ½ cup of yogurt, remaining two-thirds of the garlic, the ground chicken, bread-crumbs, egg, 1 tablespoon of olive oil, the parsley, paprika, cumin, ginger, and cin-namon. Stir to combine. You may need to use your hands here to thoroughly com-bine everything. Using a tablespoon or ice cream scoop, begin to shape the meatballs. Place them on a plate and set aside.

3. In a large skillet, heat the remaining 1 tablespoon of olive oil over medium heat. Add the meatballs, flipping them often, until they're browned and have an internal temperature of at least 165°F. You may

need to do this in batches, depending on the size of your skillet. Each batch should take 4 to 5 minutes. Transfer the cooked meatballs to a paper towel–lined plate to help absorb any excess oil.

4. To serve, spread some yogurt sauce on a plate and arrange 2 or 3 meatballs on top. Serve with the fresh arugula.

FAT LOSS: Adding Rainbow Hummus (page 160) and whole-wheat pita increase the total fiber for a complete meal to meet your goals.

PER SERVING (2 OR 3 MEATBALLS): Calories: 338; Protein: 28g; Total Carbohydrates: 13g; Fiber: 1g; Fat: 21g

---

MACROS: 31% Protein; 55% Fat; 14% Carbohydrates

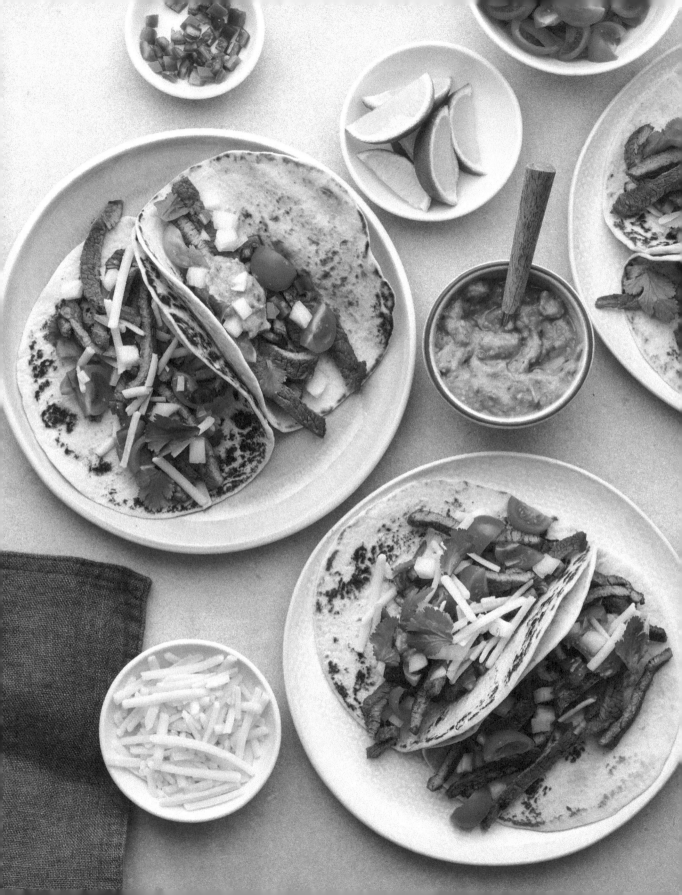

BEEF, PORK, AND LAMB MEALS

Orange-Ginger Beef

PREP TIME: 15 minutes • **COOK TIME:** 30 minutes • **SERVES 4**

If you don't have freshly squeezed orange juice for this recipe, store-bought orange juice with no pulp can also be used. This is a quick weeknight dinner that's also great for meal prep.

1½ cups quick brown rice

⅓ cup freshly squeezed orange juice, no pulp

4 garlic cloves, minced, divided

1 teaspoon minced fresh ginger

2 tablespoons low-sodium soy sauce

1 teaspoon cornstarch

2 teaspoons water

2 tablespoons olive oil, divided

12 ounces top sirloin steak, thinly sliced

1 cup ¼-inch-thick carrot slices

1 red bell pepper, seeded and thinly sliced

1 green bell pepper, seeded and thinly sliced

Salt

Freshly ground black pepper

FAT LOSS: To up the fiber in this recipe, you can omit the brown rice and replace it with additional veggies such as broccoli, green beans, or asparagus.

1. Cook the rice according to the package instructions. Set aside.

2. To make the sauce, combine the orange juice, half of the garlic, the ginger, and the soy sauce in a small saucepan and bring it to a boil over medium-high heat.

3. In a small bowl, mix the cornstarch and water. Add the mixture to the saucepan, reduce the heat to low, and stir until combined. Cook, stirring occasionally, until the marinade thickens, 6 to 8 minutes. Set aside.

4. Heat 1 tablespoon of oil in a large non-stick skillet over medium-high heat. Add the steak and cook, stirring frequently, until browned, 5 to 8 minutes. Transfer to a plate.

5. In the same skillet, heat the remaining 1 tablespoon of oil. Add the remaining half of the garlic and sauté for 1 minute. Add the carrots and cook for 4 to 5 minutes. Add the red and green bell peppers and cook until tender, 4 to 6 minutes.

CONTINUED >>

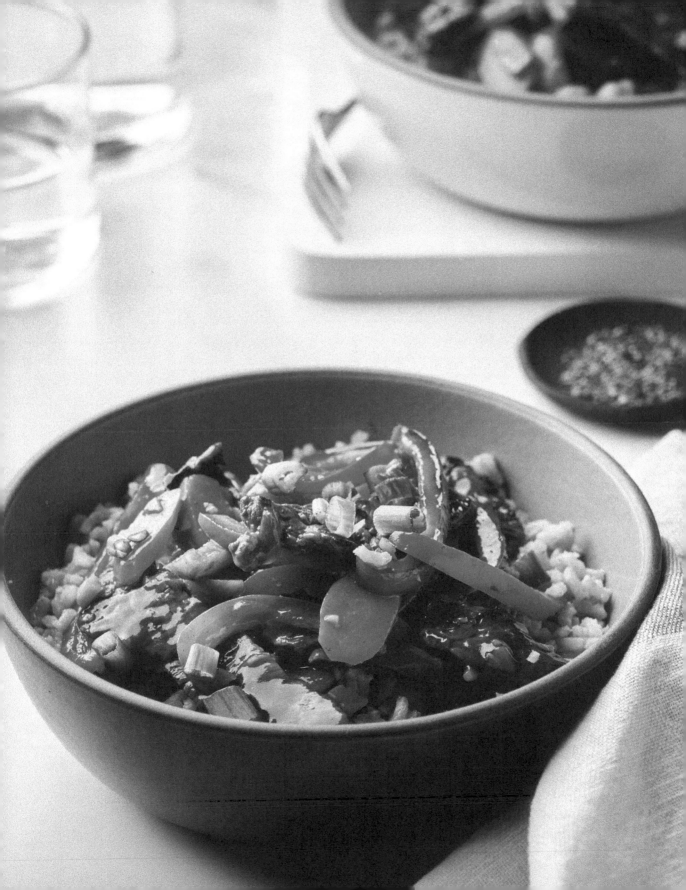

6. Add the steak and the sauce and mix well.

7. Divide the rice between four bowls. Top with the steak and sauce. Season with salt and pepper and serve. This dish will also store nicely in an airtight container in the fridge for up to 3 days.

PER SERVING (3 OZ BEEF, ⅓ CUP RICE, AND ¼ VEGETABLES): Calories: 528; Protein: 25g; Total Carbohydrates: 65g; Fiber: 5g; Fat: 18g

---

MACROS: 19% Protein; 31% Fat; 50% Carbohydrates

Beef Nacho'd Peppers

PREP TIME: 15 minutes • **COOK TIME:** 20 minutes • **SERVES 4**

Here's a take on classic nachos using a veggie chip, which increases the total fiber load, vitamin C, vitamin A, and potassium and makes this a winning macro-friendly option for a tailgate snack or game-day food. While the nachos are baking, you can even prep additional toppings, such as avocado crema, chopped onions, lime wedges, and cilantro.

Nonstick cooking spray
   (optional)
1 pound lean ground beef
1 tablespoon chili powder
1½ teaspoons ground cumin
1 tablespoon garlic powder
3 tablespoons canned chopped
   green chiles
1 (15-ounce) can black beans,
   drained and rinsed
1 (1-pound) bag mini bell
   peppers, halved
Salt
Freshly ground black pepper
1 cup shredded Mexican cheese

FAT LOSS: You can play with the meat options in this recipe. I like ground beef the best, but ground turkey or ground chicken will also work if you're looking to lower the saturated fat. Pair this with 5-Minute Guac (page 164) and you have yourself a complete meal with additional fiber.

1. Preheat the oven to 400°F. Spray a rimmed baking sheet with cooking spray or line it with aluminum foil.

2. In a large skillet over medium-high heat, brown the beef. Add the chili powder, cumin, garlic powder, and green chiles. Sauté until fully cooked, about 8 minutes. Add the black beans and cook, stirring, for 2 minutes. Remove from the heat and set aside.

3. Prep your mini bell peppers by cutting off the tops. Halve each of them and clean out the insides.

4. Place the peppers on the prepared baking sheet and season with salt and pepper. Stuff each pepper with the meat and bean mixture and sprinkle with the shredded cheese. Bake for 10 minutes.

PER SERVING (ABOUT 4 PEPPERS): Calories: 437; Protein: 37g; Total Carbohydrates: 26g; Fiber: 10g; Fat: 20g

MACROS: 34% Protein; 42% Fat; 24% Carbohydrates

Chili-Rubbed Steak Tacos

PREP TIME: 1 hour 20 minutes • **COOK TIME:** 10 minutes • **SERVES 8**

If you prep the marinade the day before, it makes this recipe quick and easy. In less than 10 minutes, these tacos will be ready to eat and enjoy. If meal-prepping, throw all the ingredients in a container, and eat like a salad or pair with tortillas.

Juice of 1 lime
2 tablespoons olive oil
2 tablespoons chili powder
3 teaspoons salt, divided
1 teaspoon garlic powder
2 pounds flank or skirt steak
16 (6-inch) tortillas,
    whole-wheat or corn, warmed

OPTIONAL TOPPINGS
5-Minute Guac (page 164) or
    store-bought
½ cup shredded Cheddar
    cheese
1 pound cherry tomatoes,
    chopped
2 jalapeño peppers, seeded and
    diced
½ cup chopped white onion
Lime wedges
Fresh cilantro

1. Whisk together the lime juice, olive oil, chili powder, 2 teaspoons of salt, and garlic powder in a baking dish or large zip-top bag. Add the steak, turning to coat it in the marinade. Cover the dish or seal the bag and let the steak marinate in the refrigerator for at least 1 hour or up to 24 hours.

2. Place the oven rack in the top position and preheat the broiler.

3. Place the steak on a rimmed baking sheet, discarding the marinade. Broil for 3 to 4 minutes per side. Transfer to a cutting board and let rest for 5 minutes. If your steak is thicker, you may need to broil it for a bit longer.

4. Thinly slice the steak and serve in the warmed tortillas with your desired toppings.

FAT LOSS: To increase the total fiber, there are several options for this recipe. Look for whole-wheat tortillas instead of corn. Keep your taco toppings veggie-forward, such as cabbage or peppers.

PER SERVING (2 TACOS): Calories: 383; Protein: 29g; Total Carbohydrates: 32g; Fiber: 2g; Fat: 15g

MACROS: 32% Protein; 34% Fat; 34% Carbohydrates

Weeknight Steak Salad

PREP TIME: 40 minutes • **COOK TIME:** 10 minutes • **SERVES 6**

This combination is perfect in the winter when you need a hearty salad, but it also fits into a busy summer routine for a high-protein, veggie-forward meal.

1½ pounds flank steak

Juice of 1 lime

1 teaspoon chili powder

½ teaspoon paprika

½ teaspoon ground cumin

½ teaspoon garlic powder

Salt

Freshly ground black pepper

6 cups greens, such as spinach or arugula

2 cups cherry tomatoes, chopped

1 avocado, peeled, pitted, and sliced

½ red onion, sliced

Blue cheese crumbles, for serving (optional)

¾ cup "Dress It Up" Salad Dressing (page 165) or store-bought (optional)

MUSCLE GAIN: This recipe is naturally lower in carbohydrates, so pairing it with a slice of whole-grain bread is a great way to add fiber-rich carbs while soaking up every bit of flavor from the dish.

1. Place the steak on a rimmed baking sheet. Squeeze the lime juice over the top.

2. In a small bowl, prep the dry rub by mixing the chili powder, paprika, cumin, garlic powder, salt, and pepper together.

3. Add the spice rub to the meat, pressing with your fingers so that it adheres. Cover and refrigerate for 30 minutes to 4 hours.

4. After the steak has marinated, heat a grill or grill pan to medium-high heat.

5. Grill the steak for 4 to 5 minutes on each side to an internal temperature of 135°F for medium-rare or 145°F for medium.

6. Transfer the steak to a cutting board and let it rest for 10 minutes. Slice thinly.

7. To assemble the salads, place the greens on a large platter. Add the sliced steak, tomatoes, avocado, and red onion. Serve blue cheese on the side for those that want it. Drizzle with dressing and enjoy!

PER SERVING (4 OZ STEAK, ⅙ VEGETABLES, AND 2 TABLESPOONS DRESSING): Calories: 313; Protein: 26g; Total Carbohydrates: 12g; Fiber: 4g; Fat: 18g

MACROS: 35% Protein; 52% Fat; 13% Carbohydrates

Stir-Fry Beef with Vegetables

PREP TIME: 15 minutes • **COOK TIME:** 15 minutes • **SERVES 4**

I love this stir-fry as a high-protein, veggie forward meal prep option. Use any of your favorite vegetables here; I like broccoli and bell peppers, as both keep their crunch when sautéed.

1 pound skirt steak, thinly sliced
2 garlic cloves, minced
1 teaspoon grated fresh ginger
Salt
Freshly ground black pepper
1 tablespoon olive oil
½ cup water
4 cups broccoli florets
1 red bell pepper, seeded and
  sliced
1 orange bell pepper, seeded
  and sliced
2 tablespoons sesame oil
½ cup low-sodium soy sauce
1 teaspoon red pepper flakes
2 teaspoons cornstarch
Dash Sriracha-Style Chile Sauce
  (page 162) or store- bought
  (optional)

MUSCLE GAIN: For added fiber, steam some brown rice and use it as a bed for the stir-fry. I suggest ½ to ¾ cup of rice to start, depending on the total carbs you're aiming to get in for this meal.

1. In a mixing bowl, combine the sliced steak, garlic, ginger, and a pinch each of salt and black pepper. Stir to combine.

2. Heat the olive oil in a large skillet over medium-high heat. Add the seasoned steak slices and cook for 4 to 5 minutes, until browned, flipping halfway through. Remove from pan. Set aside.

3. Add the water, broccoli, and bell peppers to the same skillet and cook until slightly tender, 5 to 7 minutes.

4. While the veggies are cooking, in a small bowl, whisk together the sesame oil, soy sauce, red pepper flakes, and cornstarch.

5. Once the veggies are tender, return the steak to the skillet. Add the sauce mixture and stir to combine. The sauce should start to thicken with the heat. Cook for 1 to 2 minutes, until the sauce reaches your desired consistency.

6. Serve with chile sauce (if desired).

PER SERVING (ABOUT 8 OZ): Calories: 356; Protein: 30g; Total Carbohydrates: 14g; Fiber: 4g; Fat: 20g

MACROS: 34% Protein; 51% Fat; 15% Carbohydrates

One-Pan Steak and Potatoes

PREP TIME: 15 minutes • **COOK TIME:** 30 minutes • **SERVES 4**

Red potatoes, which are loaded with fiber, B vitamins, iron, and potassium (leave the skin on for additional fiber). Add a veggie side to complement the high-protein steak.

1 pound baby red potatoes, cut into wedges

2 tablespoons olive oil, divided

1 teaspoon salt, divided

1 teaspoon freshly ground black pepper, divided

1 pound asparagus, cut into 1- to 2-inch pieces

1 pound skirt steak

1 sprig fresh rosemary, chopped

FAT LOSS: You can mix up the carbs for this recipe. I like it with potatoes. They can be baby reds as outlined above, sweet potatoes, or you could even omit the potatoes all together and go for a good crusty whole-grain bread for added fiber and grain.

1. Preheat the oven to 425°F.

2. In a large bowl, toss the potatoes with 1 tablespoon of olive oil, ½ teaspoon of salt, and ½ teaspoon of pepper. Spread the potatoes out on a rimmed baking sheet in an even layer and roast for 15 minutes.

3. In the same bowl, toss the asparagus with the remaining 1 tablespoon of olive oil, ¼ teaspoon of salt, and ¼ teaspoon of pepper.

4. After 15 minutes, remove the potatoes from the oven and give them a stir. Add the asparagus and spread everything out evenly.

5. Season the steak with the remaining salt, remaining pepper, and rosemary. Place the steak on top of the veggies. Roast for 10 to 15 minutes, until the steak is cooked through and the vegetables are tender.

6. Transfer to a platter, slice, and serve.

PER SERVING (4 OZ POTATOES AND 4 OZ STEAK):
Calories: 336; Protein: 27g; Total Carbohydrates: 20g; Fiber: 3g; Fat: 16g

MACROS: 33% Protein; 43% Fat; 24% Carbohydrates

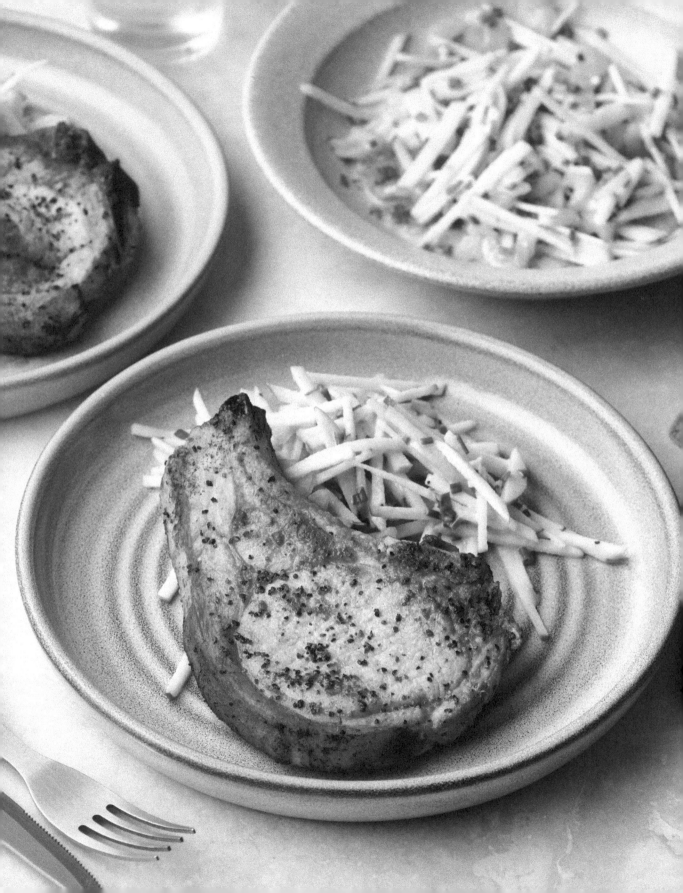

Pork Chops with Apple Slaw

PREP TIME: 15 minutes • **COOK TIME:** 15 minutes • **SERVES 4**

The apple in this recipe adds a fresh and tangy flavor to the pork. If you need a little extra spice, add some Sriracha-Style Chile Sauce from your pantry.

4 bone-in pork chops
Salt
Freshly ground black pepper
1 tablespoon olive oil
1 Honeycrisp apple
1 Gala apple
1 Granny Smith apple
¼ cup avocado mayonnaise
4 teaspoons apple cider vinegar
Dash Sriracha-Style Chile Sauce
  (page 162) or store-bought
4 celery stalks, thinly sliced
¼ cup snipped fresh chives

1. Season the pork chops with salt and pepper. Heat the oil in a large heavy-duty skillet over medium-high heat. Add the pork chops to the skillet and cook, turning occasionally, until browned with an internal temperature of 135°F, 5 to 6 minutes each side.

2. Meanwhile, cut each apple into quarters, discarding the cores. Thinly slice the quarters lengthwise, stack the slices, and then cut them again into thin sticks.

3. In a medium bowl, whisk together the mayonnaise, vinegar, and chile sauce and season with salt and pepper. Add the apple sticks, celery, and chives. Toss to combine. Serve immediately with the pork chops.

MUSCLE GAIN: For additional grains in this recipe, I love to pair it with a side of quinoa. The quinoa adds fiber, protein, and carbohydrates, making it more fitting to a Muscle Gain macro goal.

PER SERVING (1 PORK CHOP WITH ½ CUP SLAW): Calories: 378; Protein: 25g; Total Carbohydrates: 19g; Fiber: 4g; Fat: 23g

MACROS: 28% Protein; 52% Fat; 20% Carbohydrates

Sheet-Pan Sausage and Brussels Sprouts

PREP TIME: 10 minutes • **COOK TIME:** 25 minutes • **SERVES 4**

Brussels sprouts boast high levels of nutrients, including vitamin C, vitamin K, vitamin B$_6$, potassium, iron, thiamine, magnesium, and phosphorus. They also add a fiber punch, as just ½ cup contains 2 grams of fiber.

1 pound bratwurst or Italian sausage

1 pound Brussels sprouts, halved

2 tablespoons olive oil

Salt

Freshly ground black pepper

1 tablespoon honey

1 tablespoon Dijon mustard

¼ cup chopped walnuts

MUSCLE GAIN: Add whole-grain bread for extra carbohydrates, iron, and zinc. This can help you meet your post-workout carb needs.

1. Preheat the oven to 450°F. Place a rimmed baking sheet in the oven to preheat.

2. To prep the sausages, score them on both sides, being sure to not cut all the way through. In a medium bowl, toss the sausages and Brussels sprouts with the olive oil, salt, and pepper. Stir to combine.

3. Spread the sausage and sprouts out on the preheated baking sheet in an even layer. Roast for 15 minutes. To obtain a nice crunch on the Brussels sprouts, start with them cut side down.

4. Meanwhile, in a small bowl, combine the honey and mustard.

5. Drizzle the honey mustard over the sausages and sprouts and toss or shake to coat. Sprinkle with the walnuts. Roast for another 10 minutes, until the vegetables are tender.

PER SERVING (1 SAUSAGE LINK AND 4 OZ BRUSSELS SPROUTS): Calories: 567; Protein: 22g; Total Carbohydrates: 16g; Fiber: 5g; Fat: 47g

MACROS: 75% Protein; 15% Fat; 10% Carbohydrates

Sweet and Savory Grilled Pork Chops

PREP TIME: 15 minutes • **COOK TIME:** 15 minutes • **SERVES 4**

Pork, naturally a very lean meat, lends itself nicely to a variety of flavor profiles. Adding the spices in addition to the fresh mango salsa takes it to a new level in this quick recipe.

4 boneless pork chops
1 tablespoon olive oil
½ teaspoon garlic powder
½ teaspoon salt
½ teaspoon minced onion
½ teaspoon dried basil
2 ripe mangos, peeled, pitted, and diced
1 small red onion, diced
1 jalapeño pepper, seeded and diced
Juice of 1 lime
Freshly ground black pepper

MUSCLE GAIN: Look for additional carbohydrates to ensure you're meeting your carb target after a tough workout. I love this pork next to a side of black beans or even some brown rice. You can season the beans with a similar spice mixture to the one used in this recipe to bring the flavors together.

1. Rub the pork chops with the olive oil.

2. In a small bowl, combine the garlic powder, salt, minced onion, and basil. Season each side of the pork with about ¼ teaspoon of the spice mixture.

3. Heat a grill or grill pan to medium-high heat. Brush the grates with olive oil to prevent the pork chops from sticking.

4. While the grill is heating up, prep the mango salsa. In a medium bowl, combine the mangos, onion, jalapeño, and lime juice. Season with salt and pepper.

5. Once the grill is hot, grill the pork chops for 5 to 6 minutes per side. The pork is done when it reaches an internal temperature of 145°F.

6. Remove the pork from the grill and let it rest for 5 minutes.

7. Serve with the mango salsa.

PER SERVING (1 PORK CHOP WITH 2 OZ SALSA): Calories: 332; Protein: 27g; Total Carbohydrates: 31g; Fiber: 4g; Fat: 12g

MACROS: 33% Protein; 32% Fat; 35% Carbohydrates

Easy Breaded Pork Chops

PREP TIME: 15 minutes • **COOK TIME:** 25 minutes • **SERVES 4**

When using whole-wheat panko breadcrumbs for extra fiber, be sure to get a light coating, as you still want the pork to be the star.

Nonstick cooking spray

1 pound Brussels sprouts, halved

1 Gala apple, cored and cut into wedges

3 tablespoons olive oil

1 tablespoon brown sugar

¼ teaspoon dried sage

Salt

Freshly ground black pepper

4 bone-in pork chops

2 large eggs, beaten

¼ cup 1% milk or unsweetened nondairy alternative

1½ cups whole-wheat panko breadcrumbs

½ teaspoon garlic powder

¼ teaspoon onion powder

¼ teaspoon dried oregano

¼ teaspoon dried basil

¼ teaspoon dried thyme

¼ teaspoon paprika

FAT LOSS: If you want to reduce the total carbs, you can cut the amount of breadcrumbs in half, giving you a high-protein, lower-carb meal.

1. Preheat the oven to 425°F. Spray a rimmed baking sheet with cooking spray or line with aluminum foil.

2. In a large bowl, combine the Brussels sprouts, apple, olive oil, brown sugar, and sage. Season with salt and pepper. Set aside.

3. Season the pork chops with salt and pepper.

4. In a large bowl, whisk the eggs and milk. In another large bowl, whisk together the breadcrumbs, garlic powder, onion powder, oregano, basil, thyme, and paprika. Season with salt and pepper.

5. Dip each pork into the egg mixture, then dredge in the panko mixture, pressing to coat. Place each chop on the prepared baking sheet. Spread the Brussels sprout mixture around the chops.

6. Bake for 10 to 12 minutes. Turn the chops over and bake for an additional 10 minutes, or until the pork has reached a minimum internal temperature of 140°F. Serve immediately.

PER SERVING (1 PORK CHOP WITH ½ CUP BRUSSELS SPROUTS): Calories: 427; Protein: 32g; Total Carbohydrates: 30g; Fiber: 6g; Fat: 20g

MACROS: 30% Protein; 43% Fat; 27% Carbohydrates

Spiced Lamb, Brown Rice, and Hummus Bowls

PREP TIME: 10 minutes • **COOK TIME:** 15 minutes • **SERVES 4**

This lamb recipe combines the warming spices of cinnamon and allspice to create a flavorful dish that works for meal prep. Rainbow Hummus completes these bowls.

Nonstick cooking spray

1 small yellow onion, finely chopped

3 garlic cloves, minced

1 tablespoon minced fresh ginger

1 pound ground lamb

¼ cup chopped fresh mint leaves

1 teaspoon ground cinnamon

1 teaspoon ground allspice

½ teaspoon salt

¼ teaspoon red pepper flakes

3 cups cooked brown rice

1 English cucumber, chopped

2 ripe tomatoes, chopped

½ cup Rainbow Hummus (page 160) or store-bought

¼ cup feta cheese crumbles

1. Heat a large skillet over medium heat and coat with cooking spray. Add the onion and sauté for 5 minutes, until softened.

2. Add the garlic and ginger and cook for 30 seconds, until fragrant.

3. Add the lamb and cook for 5 minutes, until browned. Stir in the mint, cinnamon, allspice, salt, and red pepper flakes.

4. Divide the rice between bowls and top evenly with the lamb mixture. Top with the cucumber, tomatoes, hummus, and feta cheese.

5. Leftovers can be stored in the refrigerator for up to 3 days.

FAT LOSS: You can substitute spinach for the rice to cut back on carbs.

PER SERVING (4 OZ LAMB WITH 2 TABLESPOONS HUMMUS AND ¾ CUP RICE): Calories: 499; Protein: 31g; Total Carbohydrates: 49g; Fiber: 6g; Fat: 20g

MACROS: 24% Protein; 36% Fat; 40% Carbohydrates

Mediterranean Lamb Flatbreads

PREP TIME: 10 minutes • **COOK TIME:** 20 minutes • **SERVES 4**

Lamb is an incredible source of iron, selenium, and zinc. Look for grass-fed lamb when shopping, as the omega-3 fatty acid content tends to be a little higher in grass-fed varieties.

2 tablespoons olive oil, divided

1 garlic clove, minced

¼ cup red onion, diced

8 ounces ground lamb

1 teaspoon dried oregano

1 tablespoon fresh parsley, chopped

4 whole-wheat naan

4 ounces goat cheese, crumbled

1 cup baby spinach

2 plum tomatoes, cut into ¼-inch slices

¼ cup Macro-Friendly Pesto (page 158) or store-bought

1. Preheat the oven to 425°F.

2. In a small sauté pan, heat 1 tablespoon of olive oil over medium heat. Add the garlic and onion and sauté for about 3 minutes, or until fragrant. Add the lamb, oregano, and parsley. Sauté for 6 minutes, breaking up the ground lamb with a spatula.

3. Brush the remaining 1 tablespoon of olive oil on one side of each naan. Evenly spread the cheese, spinach, tomatoes, and lamb over each piece.

4. Bake the naan directly on the oven rack for about 8 minutes, until the crust is golden brown.

5. Drizzle the flatbreads with pesto and serve.

FAT LOSS: To lessen the total carb load, you can skip the naan and opt for a Mediterranean lamb bowl, adding hummus to the toppings for extra fiber, good fats, and iron.

PER SERVING (1 NAAN): Calories: 642; Protein: 30g; Total Carbohydrates: 52g; Fiber: 6g; Fat: 32g

MACROS: 18% Protein; 49% Fat; 33% Carbohydrates

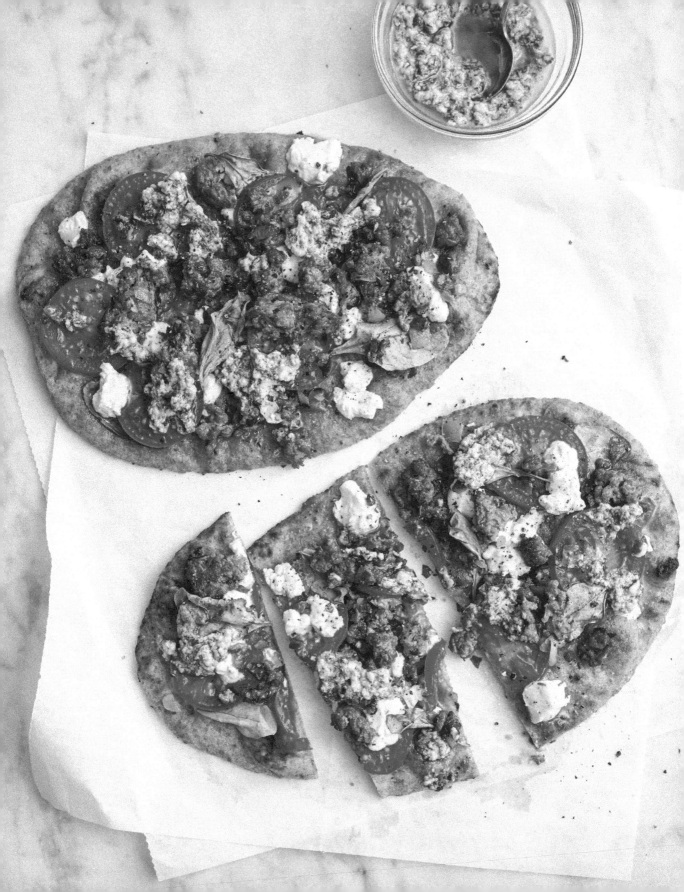

Lamb Burgers and Sweet Potato Chips

PREP TIME: 15 minutes • **COOK TIME:** 35 minutes • **SERVES 4**

Here's a twist on your basic burger and fries, with Mediterranean flavors. Couscous adds texture to the lamb burger, while the yogurt provides an added protein and calcium bump.

2 large sweet potatoes, scrubbed and cut into chips
1 tablespoon olive oil
2 teaspoons smoked paprika
½ cup water
½ cup couscous, dried
2 carrots, grated
8 ounces ground lamb
¼ cup finely chopped fresh mint
1 large egg, beaten
4 cups arugula
1 cup plain low- or nonfat Greek yogurt
Salt
Freshly ground black pepper

FAT LOSS: Portion size is an easy way you can alter this meal. If you're looking for seconds, pile on the arugula and top it with a little olive oil and balsamic vinegar for a nice salad.

1. Preheat the oven to 350°F.

2. In a large bowl, toss the potatoes with the oil. Spread the potatoes out on a rimmed baking sheet and roast for 25 minutes. Remove from the oven, season with the paprika, and roast for another 10 minutes, or until cooked through.

3. While the potatoes are roasting, bring the water to a boil in a small saucepan. Add the couscous, remove from the heat, and cover with a lid. Let the couscous sit until it has absorbed all the water, 3 to 5 minutes. Stir in the carrots, lamb, mint, and egg. Season with salt and pepper.

4. Shape the lamb mixture into 4 burgers. Heat a grill or grill pan to high heat, then grill the burgers for 6 to 8 minutes on each side.

5. Divide the chips among four plates and place a burger on each plate. Add 1 cup of arugula and ¼ cup of Greek yogurt to each plate for some extra tartness.

PER SERVING (1 BURGER AND ½ SWEET POTATO):
Calories: 355; Protein: 20g; Total Carbohydrates: 38g; Fiber: 6g; Fat: 14g

MACROS: 22% Protein; 35% Fat; 43% Carbohydrates

Macro-Friendly Lamb Tagine

PREP TIME: 15 minutes • **COOK TIME:** 1 hour 30 minutes • **SERVES 4**

Tagine is an important part of Moroccan cuisine and is cooked in a specific ceramic vessel. This stew-like dish can be made of meat, poultry, or fish and often includes veggies or fruit. Here's my take using a Dutch oven to pre-pare it. Try serving this with couscous or rice for added grains.

2 tablespoons olive oil
1 pound lamb shoulder
   or stew meat, diced
1 onion, chopped
2 large carrots, chopped
2 garlic cloves, minced
2 tablespoons garam masala
1 (15-ounce) can chopped
   tomatoes
Salt
Freshly ground black pepper
1 (15-ounce) can chickpeas,
   drained and rinsed
½ cup dried apricots, chopped
3 cups low-sodium chicken
   broth

1. Preheat the oven to 325°F.

2. In a Dutch oven, heat the olive oil over medium-high heat. Add the lamb and brown on all sides. Remove it from the skillet and set aside.

3. In the same Dutch oven, add the onion and carrots. Cook for 2 to 3 minutes, until golden. Add the garlic and cook for another minute. Stir in the garam masala and tomatoes with their juices and season with salt and pepper.

4. Return the lamb to the pot along with the chickpeas and apricots and stir to combine. Pour in the broth, stir, and bring to a simmer. Cover the dish and place in the oven for 1 hour. The lamb should be tender; if it's still tough, you can add another 20 minutes.

MUSCLE GAIN: If you need to bump up the total carbohydrates and fiber, you can add a serving of your favorite grains.

PER SERVING (8 TO 12 OZ): Calories: 374; Protein: 29g; Total Carbohydrates: 33g; Fiber: 7g; Fat: 14g

MACROS: 31% Protein; 35% Fat; 34% Carbohydrates

Lamb Meatballs with Yogurt

PREP TIME: 15 minutes • **COOK TIME:** 10 minutes • **SERVES 6**

These meatballs are filled with flavor and spice. I love to pair them with a fresh salad to keep the meal feeling light. The yogurt brings everything together with its rich creaminess.

1½ pounds ground lamb
1 small red onion, diced
1 large egg
2 garlic cloves, minced
Small handful fresh mint, chopped
1 teaspoon dried oregano
1 tablespoon olive oil, divided
Salt
Freshly ground black pepper
4 cups chopped romaine
1 large cucumber, chopped
1½ cups cherry tomatoes, halved
½ cup Kalamata olives, halved
1½ teaspoons red wine vinegar
1 tablespoon freshly squeezed lemon juice
1 cup plain low-fat or nonfat Greek yogurt
Homemade Pita Chips (page 155), for serving (optional)

1. In a large bowl, mix the lamb, onion, egg, garlic, mint, oregano, ½ tablespoon of oil, salt, and pepper. Cover and place in the refrigerator to give the flavors time to meld.

2. While the lamb is marinating, make the salad. In a serving bowl, toss the romaine with the cucumber, tomatoes, and olives. Drizzle in the red wine vinegar, remaining ½ tablespoon of oil, and lemon juice.

3. Remove the lamb mixture from the refrigerator. Using a tablespoon, scoop and roll the mixture into meatballs.

4. Warm a cast-iron skillet over medium heat. Cook the meatballs for 5 to 7 minutes, stirring occasionally, until golden brown and cooked through.

5. Plate each serving of meatballs with the salad and ¼ cup of Greek yogurt. You can also serve with pita chips for some added crunch.

MUSCLE GAIN: To add some carbohydrates, be sure to include the pita chips or pair the meatballs with couscous, a side of pasta, or even a slice of crusty bread.

PER SERVING (2 OR 3 MEATBALLS): Calories: 316; Protein: 27g; Total Carbohydrates: 9g; Fiber: 2g; Fat: 20g

MACROS: 34% Protein; 56% Fat; 10% Carbohydrates

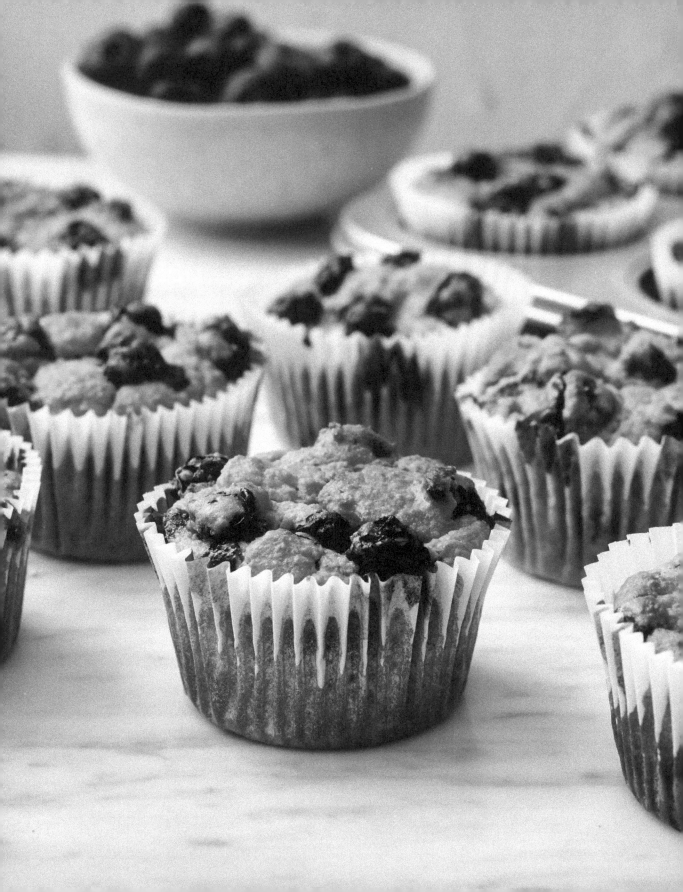

7

SNACKS AND DESSERTS

Zesty Kale Chips

PREP TIME: 10 minutes • **COOK TIME:** 15 minutes • **SERVES 6**

Crispy, full of flavor, and packed with nutrients like vitamin A, vitamin C, vitamin K, fiber, and even a bit of protein, these kale chips are seasoned with lime zest and spice to give them that extra kick to keep the party going. Get ready—these are going to go fast!

20 cups kale (2 or 3 large bunches), washed and well dried
¼ cup olive oil
1 teaspoon salt
Grated zest of 2 limes
Chili powder
Flaky sea salt

MUSCLE GAIN: For additional flavor and added protein, you can sprinkle freshly grated Parmesan cheese over the chips alongside the lime zest and chili powder. Just ¼ cup of Parmesan provides 9 grams of additional protein, plus calcium, iron, and zinc.

1. Preheat the oven to 350°F.

2. Tear the kale into bite-size pieces and place in a large bowl. You may need to work in batches depending on how large your bowl is.

3. Pour the olive oil over the kale, season with the salt, and toss to evenly distribute. The kale will be glossy. If doing this in batches, divide the olive oil accordingly.

4. Spread the kale out on two rimmed baking sheets. Bake until the leaves are crispy and ready to crumble, 13 to 16 minutes.

5. Remove from the oven and let cool. Sprinkle with the lime zest, chili powder, and flaky sea salt to taste. You can store these chips in a sealed container at room temperature for up to 3 days.

PER SERVING (1½ CUPS): Calories: 106; Protein: 2g; Total Carbohydrates: 5g; Fiber: 2g; Fat: 10g

MACROS: 5% Protein; 79% Fat; 16% Carbohydrates

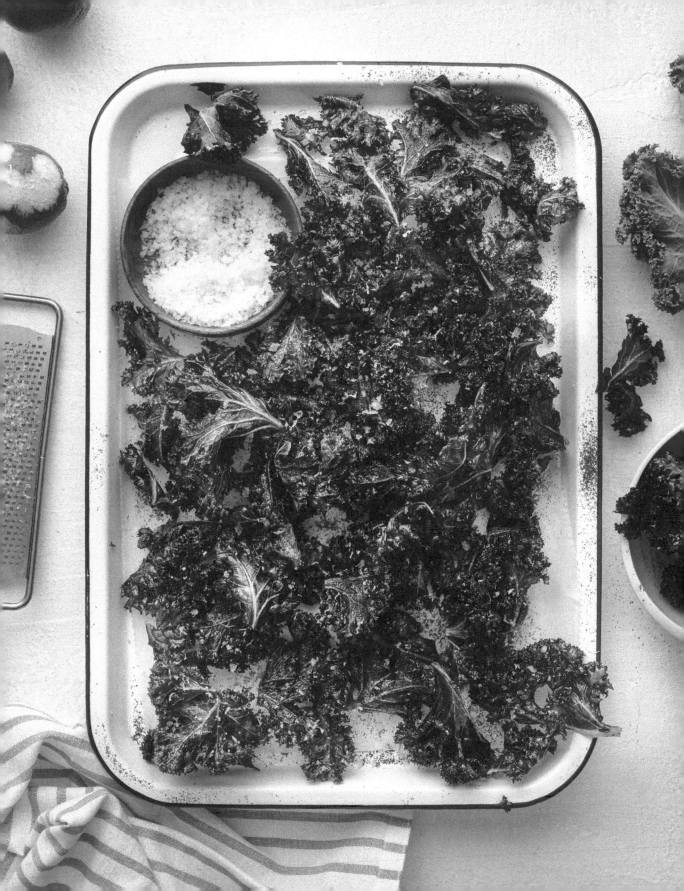

Garlic Spiced Nuts

PREP TIME: 5 minutes • **COOK TIME:** 15 minutes • **SERVES 6**

Any combination of nuts will work for this recipe, including walnuts, Brazil nuts, almonds, hazelnuts, cashews, pistachios, and pecans. During the fall, pumpkin seeds can even add a seasonal touch.

1½ teaspoons coarse sea salt
1 teaspoon ground cardamom
1 teaspoon chili powder
½ teaspoon ground turmeric
½ teaspoon garlic powder
½ teaspoon ground cinnamon
¼ teaspoon cayenne pepper
¼ teaspoon freshly ground
  black pepper
6 cups assorted raw unsalted
  nuts
2 to 3 tablespoons olive oil

1. Preheat the oven to 350°F.

2. In a small bowl, mix the salt, cardamom, chili powder, turmeric, garlic powder, cinnamon, cayenne pepper, and black pepper to combine.

3. On a rimmed baking sheet, spread the nuts out in a single layer. Drizzle with the olive oil and mix. (I start with 2 tablespoons and add another if I am unable to evenly coat the nuts.) Pour the spice mixture over the nuts and mix until evenly coated.

4. Roast for 15 minutes.

5. Remove from the oven and let cool completely. These nuts will keep in an airtight container at room temperature for up to 2 weeks or in the freezer for up to 1 month.

MUSCLE GAIN: To increase the total carbs for this snack, you can add dried fruit to make your own trail mix. This will help ensure you're meeting your energy needs post-workout.

PER SERVING (¼ CUP): Calories: 217; Protein: 6g; Total Carbohydrates: 7g; Fiber: 3g; Fat: 19g

MACROS: 9% Protein; 76% Fat; 15% Carbohydrates

Roasted Chickpeas

PREP TIME: 5 minutes • **COOK TIME:** 25 minutes • **SERVES 6**

Roasted chickpeas can be a great post-workout snack, especially after weight training. They provide protein and carbs to replenish any glycogen stores lost, along with a small amount of fat. Have these chickpeas as an appetizer before your next dinner party—the crunch, spice, and fresh flavors will win your guests over!

2 (15-ounce) cans chickpeas, rinsed, drained, and dried
2 tablespoons olive oil
1 tablespoon paprika
½ teaspoon chili powder
½ teaspoon salt
Grated zest of 1 lemon
1 sprig fresh rosemary, chopped

FAT LOSS: Use these roasted chickpeas to add fiber, protein, iron, and complex carbs to a nice green salad as your dinner entrée. If meal prepping for the week, these can make your life much simpler, as they pair nicely with almost anything.

1. Preheat the oven to 425°F.

2. On a rimmed baking sheet, spread the chickpeas out in a single layer. Roast for 10 minutes. Shake the pan, then return it to the oven and roast for another 10 minutes.

3. While the chickpeas are roasting, combine the olive oil, paprika, chili powder, salt, lemon zest, and rosemary in a large bowl.

4. Once the chickpeas are done roasting, remove them from the oven. Carefully transfer the chickpeas to the bowl with the oil mixture and toss until coated well. Return to the baking sheet and roast for another 3 to 5 minutes, until fragrant. Let cool or serve warm. Store in an airtight container in the refrigerator for up to 5 days.

PER SERVING (½ CUP): Calories: 178; Protein: 7g; Total Carbohydrates: 23g; Fiber: 7g; Fat: 7g

MACROS: 15% Protein; 33% Fat; 52% Carbohydrates

Stuffed Avocado

PREP TIME: 10 minutes • **SERVES 2**

An avocado acts as the perfect bowl for this picturesque salad. Corn and black beans make it carbohydrate-rich, while the tomato and cilantro provide a burst of color and flavor. Avocados are rich in potassium, fiber, and monounsaturated fats, making this a great snack or meal for those focusing on muscle gain and hitting high macronutrient targets.

1 (15-ounce) can black beans, drained and rinsed

1 (15-ounce) can sweet corn, drained and rinsed

1 Roma tomato, diced

2 tablespoons chopped fresh cilantro

Juice of 1 lime

1 garlic clove, minced

Pinch salt

Pinch freshly ground black pepper

1 avocado, halved and pitted

1. In a small bowl, combine the beans and corn. Add the diced tomato and cilantro and stir. Add the lime juice, garlic, salt, and pepper and mix until combined.

2. Divide the bean salad between the avocado halves and serve.

FAT LOSS: You can cut back on the black beans and corn to reduce the carbohydrates in this recipe, starting with cutting the total of each in half and seeing where that puts you on your macro counts for the day. You can also pair this with a lean protein for a complete meal.

PER SERVING (½ AVOCADO): Calories: 484; Protein: 18g; Total Carbohydrates: 77g; Fiber: 22g; Fat: 16g

MACROS: 12% Protein; 28% Fat; 60% Carbohydrates

Almond Butter Protein Bites

PREP TIME: 15 minutes • **SERVES 12**

These simple bites are naturally sweetened with dates, providing antioxidants and fiber. Dark chocolate chips make them feel more dessert-like, while the flaxseed gives them an added boost of fiber and omega-3 fatty acids.

½ **cup pitted dates**
½ **cup maple syrup**
¼ **cup almond butter**
¼ **cup ground flaxseed**
1 cup rolled oats (not instant)
2 tablespoons dark chocolate chips

1. In a food processor, combine the dates, maple syrup, almond butter, and flaxseed. Pulse to combine and break up the dates.

2. Add the oats and pulse until the dates are finely chopped. Stir in the chocolate chips.

3. Using your hands, shape the mixture into 24 balls, about 1 inch in diameter. Store in an airtight container in the refrigerator for up to 1 week or in the freezer for up to 3 months.

MUSCLE GAIN: One option to up the protein in these bites would be to add 2 scoops of protein powder in step 1, giving these a protein bump of 4 more grams per bite. Play around with protein powder flavors, as unflavored, chocolate, or vanilla could all work.

PER SERVING (2 BITES): Calories: 130; Protein: 3g; Total Carbohydrates: 20g; Fiber: 3g; Fat: 5g

MACROS: 8% Protein; 32% Fat; 60% Carbohydrates

Anytime Granola Bars

PREP TIME: 5 minutes • **COOK TIME:** 35 minutes • **SERVES 16**

Granola bars are an easy snack on the go, but many store-bought varieties are packed with added sugars and trans fats. This is my take on a granola bar that you can take anywhere and know every ingredient that goes into it.

Nonstick cooking spray
1 tablespoon canola oil
2 cups rolled oats (not instant)
½ cup ground flaxseed
¾ teaspoon ground cinnamon
Pinch salt
¼ cup almond butter
¼ cup honey
1 tablespoon brown sugar
1 teaspoon vanilla extract
½ cup dark chocolate chips

MUSCLE GAIN: To raise the carbs in these bars, try adding dried fruit, such as raisins, dried cherries, or apricots. Start with a ½ cup of your fruit of choice, chopped, and add it alongside the chocolate chips.

1. Preheat the oven to 300°F. Grease a 9-inch square baking dish with nonstick spray.

2. Heat the oil in a medium saucepan over medium heat. Add the oats and cook for 5 to 7 minutes, stirring, until the oats start to brown and smell toasted. Transfer to a medium bowl. Add the flaxseed, cinnamon, and salt.

3. In the same saucepan, combine the almond butter, honey, brown sugar, and vanilla. Bring to a boil over medium heat, stirring occasionally. Remove from the heat and pour over the oat mixture. Stir until the oats are evenly coated. Allow to cool for 5 minutes. Stir in the chocolate chips.

4. Transfer the mixture to the prepared baking dish and spread into an even layer. You may need to use your hands or the back of a spatula to really press it down. Bake for 18 to 20 minutes, until lightly browned. Cut into 16 bars. Store in an airtight container at room temperature for up to 3 weeks.

PER SERVING (1 BAR): Calories: 138; Protein: 3g; Total Carbohydrates: 16g; Fiber: 2g; Fat: 7g

MACROS: 9% Protein; 46% Fat; 45% Carbohydrates

Blueberry–Peanut Butter Muffins

PREP TIME: 10 minutes • **COOK TIME:** 20 minutes • **SERVES 12**

This recipe uses peanut butter powder and Greek yogurt to create a high-protein blueberry muffin reminiscent of a peanut butter and jelly sandwich. For the peanut butter powder, you can substitute 2 tablespoons of peanut or almond butter—just know that this will increase the fat content, so you'll need to account for that in your final macro counts.

1 cup plain low- or nonfat Greek yogurt

½ cup unsweetened applesauce

⅓ cup maple syrup

¼ cup 1% or 2% milk or unsweetened nondairy alternative

2 tablespoons avocado oil

2 large eggs

2 cups oat flour

¼ cup peanut butter powder

1 teaspoon baking powder

1 cup fresh or frozen blueberries

1. Preheat the oven to 350°F. Line a 12-cup muffin tin with paper or silicone liners.

2. In a large bowl, combine the yogurt, applesauce, maple syrup, milk, oil, and eggs.

3. Add the oat flour, peanut butter powder, and baking powder and mix well.

4. Fold in the blueberries.

5. Spoon the batter evenly into the muffin liners. Bake for 20 minutes, or until a toothpick inserted in the center of the muffins comes out clean.

FAT LOSS: To increase total fiber, you can use whole-wheat flour in place of the oat flour.

PER SERVING (1 MUFFIN): Calories: 183; Protein: 6g; Total Carbohydrates: 22g; Fiber: 3g; Fat: 8g

MACROS: 12% Protein; 40% Fat; 48% Carbohydrates

Coconut Kettle Corn

PREP TIME: 5 minutes • **COOK TIME:** 10 minutes • **SERVES 6**

Popcorn is a comfort food to many, usually associated with loads of butter and salt. This version contains no added saturated fats, making it a whole-grain snack that's rich in fiber and low in calories.

1 tablespoon coconut oil
¼ cup popcorn kernels
1 tablespoon honey
Ground cinnamon
Salt

1. In a wide saucepan with a tight-fitting lid, heat the oil over medium-high heat. Once the oil is hot, test the temperature by dropping in 2 or 3 popcorn kernels. Wait for the kernels to pop. Once they've popped, you can add the remaining kernels. Cover with a lid and let the magic happen.

2. The kernels will pop for 3 to 4 minutes. Once the popping stops, remove the pan from the heat.

3. While the popcorn is still hot, add the honey, cinnamon, and salt. Toss to combine.

MUSCLE GAIN: This kettle corn is a great addition to your normal movie night, and one you know will not wreck your entire day of counting macros. You can boost the protein and round out the snack by adding nuts—kind of like caramel corn but without the excess sugar.

PER SERVING (1 CUP): Calories: 61; Protein: 1g; Total Carbohydrates: 9g; Fiber: 1g; Fat: 3g

MACROS: 5% Protein; 37% Fat; 58% Carbohydrates

Dessert Hummus

PREP TIME: 10 minutes • **SERVES 6**

Dessert hummus is a family favorite at our house as an after-dinner snack. Try dipping your favorite pieces of fruit (such as strawberries, apple slices, and frozen banana chips), pita chips, graham crackers, or pretzels.

1 (15-ounce) can chickpeas, drained and rinsed
⅓ cup almond butter
3 tablespoons cocoa powder
1 tablespoon maple syrup
2 tablespoons water, plus more as needed
1 teaspoon vanilla extract
Pinch salt

1. In a food processor, combine the chickpeas, almond butter, cocoa powder, maple syrup, water, vanilla, and salt and blend until smooth. You may need to periodically stop to scrape down the sides. If the mixture appears too thick, you can add additional water until it reaches reach your desired consistency.

2. Store in an airtight container in the refrigerator for up to 5 days.

FAT LOSS: This dessert is already a great source of fiber and protein, so being selective on the items you choose to dip in it will help you hit your goals. Fruits are always a healthy choice, as they're high in fiber, vitamins, and minerals and they pair great with chocolate.

PER SERVING (2 TABLESPOONS): Calories: 153; Protein: 6g; Total Carbohydrates: 15g; Fiber: 5g; Fat: 9g

MACROS: 13% Protein; 49% Fat; 38% Carbohydrates

Deconstructed Peach Pie

PREP TIME: 30 minutes • **COOK TIME:** 15 minutes • **SERVES 4**

This deconstructed pie is quick, easy, and delicious. I like to use coconut oil, rich in natural medium-chain triglycerides, for its anti-inflammatory and antioxidant properties. Any fruit "filling" can work in this recipe, including pears, berries, and apples.

⅓ cup all-purpose flour

¼ cup plus 1½ tablespoons brown sugar, divided

¼ teaspoon baking powder

2½ teaspoons ground cinnamon, divided

Pinch salt

6 tablespoons coconut oil, divided

¼ cup rolled oats (not instant)

3 large peaches, pitted and cut into ¼-inch slices (crisp ones work well)

1½ tablespoons granulated sugar

¼ teaspoon ground nutmeg

1. Preheat the oven to 375°F. Line a rimmed baking sheet with parchment paper.

2. To make the topping, whisk together the flour, ¼ cup of brown sugar, the baking powder, ½ teaspoon of cinnamon, and the salt. Add 3 tablespoons of coconut oil and use your fingers to form the mixture into pea-size balls. Add the oats and continue to form clumps. Chill the mixture for 15 minutes.

3. While the topping is chilling, in a medium bowl, combine the peaches, the remaining 1½ tablespoons of brown sugar, the granulated sugar, the remaining 2 teaspoons of cinnamon, and the nutmeg. Set aside.

4. Remove the chilled topping from the refrigerator and spread it out on the prepared baking sheet. Bake for 8 minutes, then let it cool.

5. In a large skillet, heat the remaining 3 tablespoons of coconut oil over medium heat. Add the peach mixture and sauté for 4 to 5 minutes, until browned but still tender. You may need to do this in batches, as you want the peaches in a single layer when sautéing.

6. Once the peaches are done, remove them from the heat. Serve warm with the crumble topping.

FAT LOSS: The carb load in this recipe is rather elevated, so to cut back on total carbohydrates, you can omit the added sugars in step 4. The natural sugars in the fruit will provide plenty of caramelization.

PER SERVING (ABOUT ¾ CUP): Calories: 379; Protein: 3g; Total Carbohydrates: 48g; Fiber: 4g; Fat: 21g

MACROS: 3% Protein; 48% Fat; 49% Carbohydrates

You-Pick-It Fruit Bake

PREP TIME: 10 minutes • **COOK TIME:** 45 minutes • **SERVES 6**

I like berries for this recipe, but any fresh fruit will work for this pleasing dessert with a light, bread-like crust. Let it bake while you eat dinner, and voilà, dessert is ready!

Nonstick cooking spray
6 cups sliced fresh fruit
½ cup plus 1 tablespoon brown sugar, divided
½ cup unsalted butter or coconut oil and ¼ cup softened and ¼ cup melted
1 tablespoon vanilla extract
¾ cup whole-wheat flour
1 teaspoon baking powder
Pinch flaky salt

1. Preheat the oven to 350°F. Spray a loaf pan with nonstick spray.

2. In the loaf pan, combine the fruit, ½ cup of brown sugar, ¼ cup of softened butter, and the vanilla. Toss well to combine.

3. In a small bowl, combine the flour, ½ cup of melted butter, baking powder, remaining 1 tablespoon of brown sugar, and the salt. Mix with a fork. Pour over the mixture in the loaf pan.

4. Bake for 45 minutes, or until golden brown on top. Store in the refrigerator, covered, for up to 1 week.

FAT LOSS: Pairing this dessert with protein will finish your meal in style. I like adding either creamy Greek yogurt or ricotta cheese for a little tanginess and to balance out the total carb, fat, and protein levels, better meeting both fat loss and muscle gain goals. One cup of ricotta will provide an additional 28 grams of protein.

PER SERVING (1 [1½-INCH] SLICE): Calories: 315; Protein: 3g; Total Carbohydrates: 48g; Fiber: 4g; Fat: 16g

MACROS: 3% Protein; 42% Fat; 55% Carbohydrates

One-Bowl Oatmeal–Chocolate Chip Cookies

PREP TIME: 10 minutes • **COOK TIME:** 20 minutes • **SERVES 20**

Oatmeal–chocolate chip cookies are a fan-favorite everywhere you go. Adding a healthier spin with whole-wheat flour for additional fiber, coconut oil for medium-chain triglycerides, and dark chocolate chips for an antioxidant boost, this recipe takes a beloved dessert and makes it that much better.

1¼ cups rolled oats (not instant)
1 cup whole-wheat flour
½ cup brown sugar
¼ cup granulated sugar
½ teaspoon baking soda
½ teaspoon salt
½ cup melted coconut oil
1 large egg
1½ teaspoons vanilla extract
1 cup dark chocolate chips

MUSCLE GAIN: To increase the protein in this dessert, add ½ cup of chopped walnuts in step 2 when you stir in the chocolate chips. That will raise the protein by 6 grams for the whole batch.

1. Preheat the oven to 350°F. Line a rimmed baking sheet with parchment paper.

2. In a large bowl, combine the oats, flour, brown sugar, granulated sugar, baking soda, salt, oil, egg, and vanilla. Mix with a wooden spoon or electric mixer until the dough is combined. It may be crumbly—that's okay. Fold in the chocolate chips with a wooden spoon or spatula.

3. Using a spoon, scoop about 1 tablespoon of dough and roll into a ball. If the mixture is too crumbly, you can add an additional 1 tablespoon of coconut oil.

4. Place the rolled cookies on the prepared baking sheet 2 inches apart. Bake for 15 to 20 minutes, or until golden brown. Serve warm or store in an airtight container for up to 1 week.

PER SERVING (1 COOKIE): Calories: 172; Protein: 2g; Total Carbohydrates: 18g; Fiber: 1g; Fat: 10g

MACROS: 6% Protein; 50% Fat; 44% Carbohydrates

Quinoa-Apple Crumble

PREP TIME: 15 minutes • **COOK TIME:** 1 hour 10 minutes • **SERVES 8**

I like to use a crisp apple for this dessert, like Honeycrisp or Granny Smith. Both hold up in terms of texture while providing a delicious flavor, and you can leave the skin on for added fiber and color. The oats and quinoa here provide the protein.

Nonstick cooking spray

1¼ cups rolled oats
   (not instant)

½ cup quinoa

⅓ cup plus 2 tablespoons
   brown sugar, divided

1¼ teaspoons ground
   cinnamon, divided

Pinch salt

6 tablespoons unsalted butter,
   chilled, cut into ½-inch pieces

4 or 5 large apples (about
   2½ pounds), cored and
   thinly sliced

1 tablespoon freshly squeezed
   lemon juice

¼ teaspoon ground nutmeg

1 teaspoon vanilla extract

1. Preheat the oven to 350°F. Line a rimmed baking sheet with parchment paper. Spray an 8-inch square baking dish with non-stick spray.

2. Combine the oats, quinoa, ⅓ cup of brown sugar, ¼ teaspoon of cinnamon, and the salt in a food processor. Pulse several times until combined. Add the butter and pulse until the butter is evenly distributed among the grains and the mixture has a crumbly consistency.

3. Spread the topping out on the prepared baking sheet in an even layer. Bake for 10 minutes, stir, then bake for another 5 to 10 minutes, until nicely browned. Remove from the oven and allow to cool. Increase the oven temperature to 375°F.

4. In a large bowl, toss the apple slices with the lemon juice, the remaining 2 tablespoons of brown sugar, the remaining 1 teaspoon of cinnamon, the nutmeg, and vanilla.

5. Transfer the apple mixture to the prepared baking dish and bake for 30 minutes, stirring every 10 minutes, until the apples are tender. Remove from the oven.

6. Top the baked apples with the crumble topping and return to the oven. Bake for 15 to 20 minutes, until nicely browned. Allow to cool for 10 minutes before serving.

MUSCLE GAIN: This dessert is naturally sweet from the apples. If you want to limit the amount of added sugar, you can cut back on the sugar you add to the apples and in the topping. To take the protein up a notch, I serve plain Greek yogurt as a base to top with the delicious crumble.

PER SERVING (ABOUT ⅔ CUP): Calories: 266; Protein: 4g; Total Carbohydrates: 41g; Fiber: 5g; Fat: 10g

MACROS: 5% Protein; 34% Fat; 61% Carbohydrates

Macro-Friendly Strawberry Shortcake Nice Cream

PREP TIME: 10 minutes • **SERVES 2**

Strawberry shortcake is a beloved dessert, but one that tends to be high in unwanted saturated fats. In this "nice cream" version, frozen bananas (which should be sliced before freezing) deliver a unique consistency and flavor while making for a healthier go-to treat.

2 large bananas, sliced and frozen

2 tablespoons 1% milk or unsweetened nondairy alternative

1½ cups strawberries, stemmed and halved

6 graham crackers, divided

1. In a food processor, combine the bananas and milk and pulse until smooth and creamy. Add the strawberries and 4 graham crackers. Continue to pulse until well combined.

2. Divide the mixture between two bowls. Break the remaining 2 graham crackers into small pieces, sprinkle over the top, and serve.

FAT LOSS: You can cut back on the carbs in this recipe a few different ways, such as using one banana instead of two, using Greek yogurt instead of milk, and reducing the total graham cracker amount to 3 instead of 6.

PER SERVING (ABOUT ¾ CUP): Calories: 213; Protein: 3g; Total Carbohydrates: 46g; Fiber: 6g; Fat: 3g

MACROS: 6% Protein; 14% Fat; 80% Carbohydrates

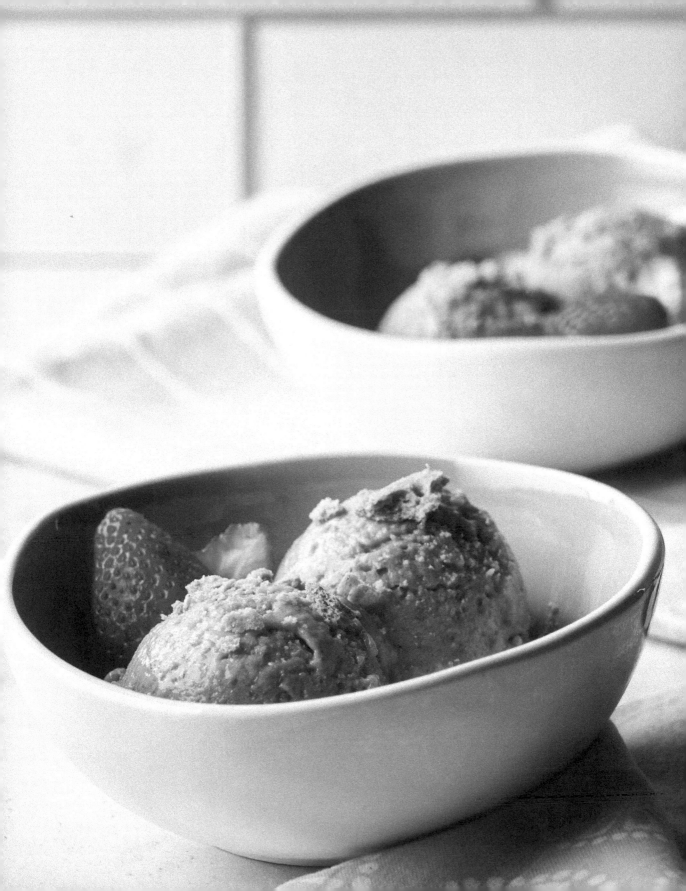

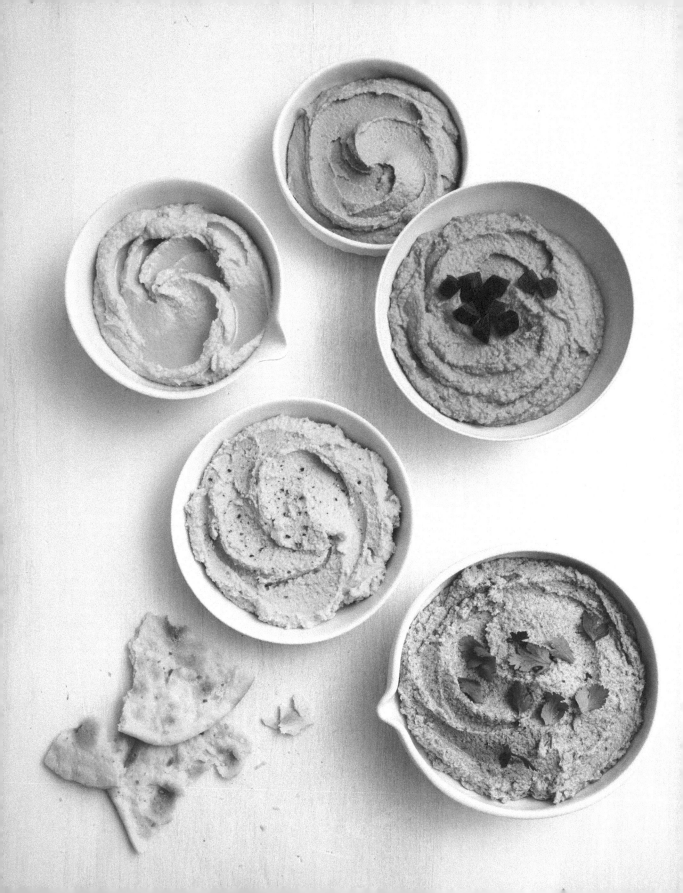

8

HOMEMADE STAPLES

Perfect Granola

PREP TIME: 5 minutes • **COOK TIME:** 30 minutes • **SERVES 12**

Granola can be a great nutrient-dense snack with lots of fast-acting carbs to refuel you after a workout, and it's easy to pack along for hikes, picnics, soccer games—you name it. Store-bought granola tends to be high in sugar and high-fructose corn syrup. By making it yourself, you'll know all the ingredients in this one!

Nonstick cooking spray

3 cups rolled oats (not instant)

1 cup walnuts, chopped

1 cup unsweetened coconut flakes

½ cup dried tart cherries, blueberries, or cranberries

¼ cup flaxseed

Pinch salt

Pinch ground cinnamon

½ cup maple syrup

½ cup coconut oil

1 teaspoon vanilla extract

1. Preheat the oven to 300°F. Spray a rimmed baking sheet with nonstick spray.

2. In a large bowl, combine the oats, walnuts, coconut, cherries, flaxseed, salt, and cinnamon. Mix well.

3. In a small saucepan over medium heat, melt together the maple syrup, coconut oil, and vanilla. Once melted, pour the warm syrup over the oat mixture and mix well.

4. Spread the granola mixture out on the prepared baking sheet and bake for 15 minutes. Remove from the oven, stir, and return to the oven. Bake for another 15 minutes, until golden brown. Granola can be stored in an airtight container at room temperature for up to 2 weeks.

FAT LOSS: To balance out the carb load in this granola and better hit your macros, pair this with your favorite Greek yogurt or cottage cheese.

PER SERVING (½ CUP): Calories: 334; Protein: 6g; Total Carbohydrates: 28g; Fiber: 5g; Fat: 22g

MACROS: 6% Protein; 56% Fat; 38% Carbohydrates

Homemade Pita Chips

PREP TIME: 5 minutes • **COOK TIME:** 15 minutes • **SERVES 4**

Crunchy pita chips can really complete a meal, and it's simple to make a double or triple batch for easy dinner prep later in the week. I've even used this recipe base to make dessert pita chips, replacing the garlic and salt with cinnamon and sugar.

4 whole-wheat pitas, cut into wedges
¼ cup coconut oil, melted
1 garlic clove, minced
Salt

1. Preheat the oven to 350°F.

2. Put the pita wedges in a large bowl. In a small bowl, whisk together the coconut oil and garlic. Pour the oil mixture over the pita and toss to gently coat. Spread the wedges out on a large baking sheet in a single layer. Sprinkle with salt.

3. Bake for 10 to 15 minutes, or until golden brown, tossing the chips partway through to ensure balanced browning. Remove from the oven and allow to cool. Store the chips in an airtight container at room temperature for up to 5 days.

MUSCLE GAIN: Pair these pita chips with any meal or snack to help you meet those carbohydrate goals and refuel and repair for the next workout.

PER SERVING (1 PITA OR 16 TO 20 CHIPS): Calories: 290; Protein: 6g; Total Carbohydrates: 35g; Fiber: 5g; Fat: 15g

MACROS: 8% Protein; 45% Fat; 47% Carbohydrates

Perfect Hard-Boiled Eggs

PREP TIME: 5 minutes • **COOK TIME:** 15 minutes • **MAKES 6 EGGS**

Hard-Boiled eggs are an excellent snack to have on hand, and this recipe is tried and true. You can play with the total cook time to reach the perfect hard-boiled egg for you.

6 large eggs

1. Place the eggs in a medium pot and cover with cold water by 1 inch.

2. Bring to a boil, then cover. Turn the heat off, but do not remove the pot from the stove. Allow the eggs to cook, covered, for 9 to 12 minutes; 9 minutes will result in a soft-boiled egg, while 12 minutes will be a hard-boiled egg.

3. Once the desired amount of time has passed, remove the eggs from the pot and place them in a bowl of ice water. Allow to cool for 10 to 15 minutes. Peel and enjoy!

4. Unpeeled eggs can be stored in the refrigerator for up to 1 week.

FAT LOSS: Filled with lean protein and nearly zero carbs, eggs are an easy add-in for when you need to bump up your protein intake. Place on top of a salad, pair them with your favorite breakfast foods, or even throw them into a veggie-filled noodle bowl.

PER SERVING (1 EGG): Calories: 72; Protein: 6g; Total Carbohydrates: 0.5g; Fiber: 0g; Fat: 5g

MACROS: 38% Protein; 60% Fat; 2% Carbohydrates

Creamy Peanut Butter

PREP TIME: 5 minutes • **MAKES 2 CUPS**

Peanut butter is one of the foods I would take with me to a deserted island. You can pair it with fruits or add it to smoothies or overnight oats to balance out the nutrient profile. While store-bought varieties tend to be packed with sugar, corn syrup, and other ingredients that don't need to be there, this homemade version is simple and clean.

⅓ **cup olive oil, plus more as needed**
¼ **cup honey (optional)**
3 cups peanuts (I like lightly salted varieties)

Feel free to use alternative oils, such as coconut oil, in place of the olive oil. The oil choice may impact the flavor profile.

1. Pour the oil and honey (if using) into a blender or food processor. Then add the peanuts.

2. Blend on high speed until it reaches your desired consistency (creamy versus crunchy). If the mixture appears thick, you can add additional oil, 1 tablespoon at a time.

3. Transfer to a glass jar and seal tightly. Store at room temperature for 1 week or in the refrigerator for up to 1 month.

FAT LOSS: If you are trying to limit your total carbohydrate intake, omit the honey.

PER SERVING (2 TABLESPOONS): Calories: 207; Protein: 7g; Total Carbohydrates: 8g; Fiber: 2g; Fat: 17g

MACROS: 12% Protein; 78% Fat; 10% Carbohydrates

Macro-Friendly Pesto

PREP TIME: 5 minutes • **MAKES ¾ CUP**

Basil is the herb used traditionally in pesto, but you can mix it up by using arugula for a nice peppery version from time to time. This easy pesto uses a combination of water and oil, but if you need more fat to hit your daily goal, use only oil.

2 cups packed fresh basil or arugula

¼ cup shredded Parmesan cheese

1 tablespoon olive oil

3 garlic cloves, peeled

2 to 3 tablespoons water

½ teaspoon salt

1. In a food processor, combine the basil, Parmesan, oil, and garlic. Pulse several times, until the mixture is roughly chopped.

2. Stream in the water as you blend. The mixture will come together to form a sauce. Season with salt and enjoy!

3. Pesto will keep in an airtight container in the refrigerator for up to 5 days or in the freezer for up to 3 months (you can even portion it out in an ice cube tray).

MUSCLE GAIN: For more protein, healthy fat, and texture, you can add walnuts or pine nuts to your pesto. Throw in ¼ cup in step 1 and watch it transform. Adding ¼ cup of pine nuts will boost the protein by 5 grams.

PER SERVING (3 TABLESPOONS): Calories: 74; Protein: 3g; Total Carbohydrates: 2g; Fiber: 0g; Fat: 6g

MACROS: 14% Protein; 74% Fat; 12% Carbohydrates

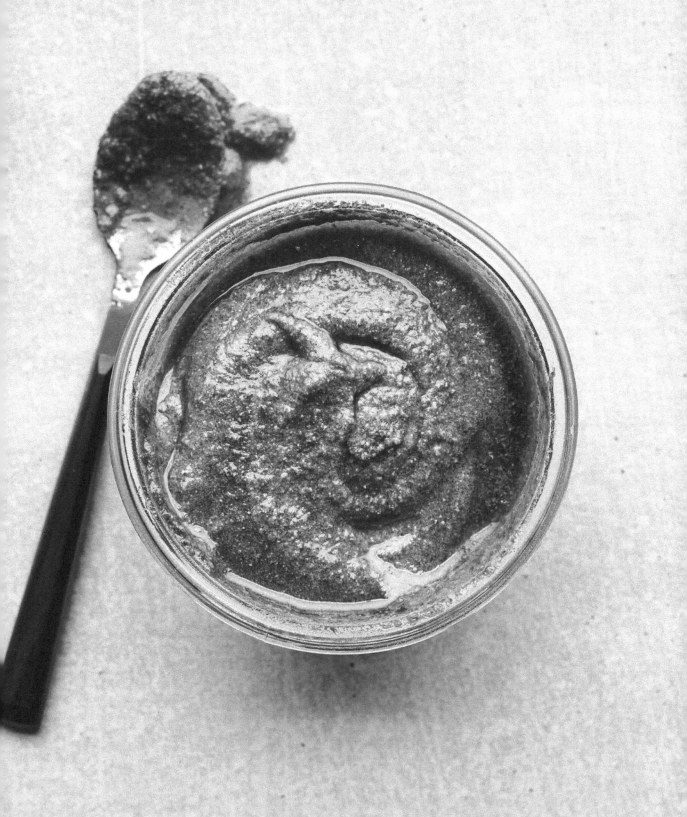

Rainbow Hummus

PREP TIME: 10 minutes • **SERVES 4**

Hummus is tangy and nutrient dense, and it pairs with most spices, herbs, and vegetables in both sweet and savory recipes. These variations transform basic hummus into bright, lively hues with added nutritional benefits in each. Pair with a meal, serve as a dip with fresh veggies, or make a beautiful food board.

1 (15-ounce) can chickpeas, drained and rinsed
2 tablespoons olive oil
¼ cup tahini
Juice of 1 lemon
1 garlic clove, peeled
¼ teaspoon salt

COLOR VARIATIONS
Pink Hummus: Add 2 ounces roasted, peeled beets.
Yellow Hummus: Add 1 teaspoon ground turmeric.
Green Hummus: Add 1 cup each fresh cilantro and parsley.
Blue Hummus: Add ½ teaspoon powdered spirulina.

1. Combine the chickpeas, olive oil, tahini, lemon juice, garlic, and salt in a food processor or blender. Add your choice of color variation and blend until smooth.

2. Store in an airtight container in the refrigerator for up to 1 week.

MUSCLE GAIN: You should tag this page now. I reference it several times throughout this book as a perfect add-on to complete a meal. Hummus is delicious, versatile, and jam-packed with nutrients. If you want to make it even more protein-packed, you can double the amount of tahini in the recipe, adding another 5 grams of protein. Pair with Homemade Pita Chips (page 155), a lean protein, and veggies and you have yourself a healthy high-protein meal.

PER SERVING (¼ CUP OF BASE RECIPE): Calories: 254; Protein: 8g; Total Carbohydrates: 21g; Fiber: 6g; Fat: 16g

MACROS: 11% Protein; 56% Fat; 33% Carbohydrates

Macro-Friendly Marinara Sauce

PREP TIME: 10 minutes • **COOK TIME:** 20 minutes • **MAKES 3½ CUPS**

Many store-bought tomato sauces are high in sugar and other additives to help with preservation. This marinara delivers not only nutrition, but home-made Italian appeal.

1 (28-ounce) can whole San
   Marzano tomatoes
¼ cup olive oil
4 garlic cloves, minced
Pinch red pepper flakes
1 teaspoon salt
1 teaspoon dried oregano

1. Pour the tomatoes and their juices into a large bowl. Use your hands to fully crush the tomatoes.

2. In a large skillet, heat the olive oil over medium heat. Add the garlic and cook until fragrant, about 30 seconds.

3. Add the tomatoes, red pepper flakes, salt, and oregano and stir.

4. Simmer until the sauce begins to thicken, about 15 minutes.

5. Store in an airtight container in the refrigerator for up to 1 week or in the freezer for up to 3 months.

MUSCLE GAIN: Pair this marinara sauce with a high-fiber, high-protein meal, such as whole-wheat pasta or veggie noodles with some meatballs (or left-over protein), plus a big salad on the side.

PER SERVING (½ CUP): Calories: 89; Protein: 1g; Total Carbohydrates: 5g; Fiber: 2g; Fat: 8g

MACROS: 3% Protein; 79% Fat; 18% Carbohydrates

Sriracha-Style Chile Sauce

PREP TIME: 5 minutes • **COOK TIME:** 10 minutes • **MAKES 1 CUP**

This chili sauce adds a nice spice to meals, without the added sugar found in many store-bought varieties. For those who like things spicy, play around with different peppers to find the heat level you like the best. I recommend wearing latex gloves when handling the chiles, as the residue is hard to get off with hand washing. Be careful not to touch your eyes!

2 chile peppers (such as habanero), chopped

1 red bell pepper, seeded and chopped

3 garlic cloves, chopped

½ cup white vinegar

½ teaspoon salt

1. Combine the chiles, bell pepper, garlic, vinegar, and salt in a small saucepan over medium heat. Bring the mixture to a simmer, reduce the heat to low, and cover. Continue to simmer, covered, until the peppers are tender, 7 to 10 minutes.

2. Transfer the mixture to a blender and blend until smooth. Pour into a glass jar and allow to cool, uncovered.

3. Once the sauce has cooled, cover tightly with a lid and store in the refrigerator for up to 6 months.

MUSCLE GAIN: This is a condiment that can boost any flavor profile. If focusing on a muscle gain goal, use this sauce on high-protein foods such as eggs, tacos, fish, meats, and poultry.

PER SERVING (1 TABLESPOON): Calories: 5; Protein: 0g; Total Carbohydrates: 1g; Fiber: 0g; Fat: 0g

MACROS: 12% Protein; 6% Fat; 82% Carbohydrates

Macro-Friendly Ketchup

PREP TIME: 10 minutes • **COOK TIME:** 25 minutes • **MAKES 1 CUP**

Ketchup is a condiment that goes with just about anything, and this tasty version is free of the excessive sugar and sodium found in store-bought versions.

2 pints grape tomatoes, halved
1 cup red wine vinegar
¼ cup brown sugar
2 teaspoons salt
1 teaspoon freshly ground black pepper
½ teaspoon Worcestershire sauce

1. In a large skillet, bring the tomatoes, vinegar, sugar, salt, and pepper to a gentle boil over medium heat. Reduce the heat and simmer until the mixture becomes jam-like and the liquid begins to evaporate, 20 to 25 minutes.

2. Transfer the mixture to a blender and blend until smooth.

3. If you want to make this ketchup very smooth, strain the mixture through a fine-mesh sieve once or twice.

4. Stir in the Worcestershire sauce.

5. Transfer to a glass jar, seal tightly, and store in the refrigerator for up to 6 months.

MUSCLE GAIN: This ketchup can fit in both fat loss– and muscle gain–oriented diets. Feel free to omit or reduce the amount of brown sugar if you are looking to decrease the total amount of carbs or want a less sweet option. The main tip here is to focus on what you're using the ketchup on. For muscle gain goals, focus on high-protein foods such as eggs, beef, and chicken.

PER SERVING (2 TABLESPOONS): Calories: 41; Protein: 1g; Total Carbohydrates: 9g; Fiber: 1g; Fat: 0g

MACROS: 5% Protein; 4% Fat; 91% Carbohydrates

5-Minute Guac

PREP TIME: 5 minutes • **SERVES 6**

*This is a simple, quick, and delicious recipe for guacamole, the side that so
many of us adore. It goes with anything: eggs, tacos, toast, veggies, and of
course, tortilla chips. With freshly squeezed lime juice and cilantro, it makes
a refreshing side.*

3 large avocados, peeled
 and pitted

3 garlic cloves, minced

½ small red onion, diced

1 medium tomato, diced

Juice of 1 lime

½ teaspoon salt

1 tablespoon chopped fresh
 cilantro

1 jalapeño pepper, seeded
 and diced (optional)

1. Scoop the avocado flesh into a medium
 bowl. Using a fork, mash the avocado
 until smooth.

2. Add the garlic, onion, tomato, lime juice,
 salt, cilantro, and jalapeño (if using).
 Mix until combined. Taste and add salt
 or additional lime juice to get the flavor
 you prefer.

3. While this is best enjoyed immediately, if
 you store it, find an airtight container and
 keep one or two avocado pits in there as
 well. The pits can help prevent further oxi-
 dation from occurring, keeping your guac
 from browning. Store in the refrigerator for
 up to 3 days.

MUSCLE GAIN: Avocados are naturally high in fiber,
making this snack a go-to for fat loss. To increase total
carbohydrates and protein, focus on the types of foods
you're putting the guacamole on, such as Blackened
Fish Tacos (page 91), Beef Nacho'd Peppers (page 115),
or Halloumi Fajitas (page 80).

PER SERVING (¼ CUP): Calories: 171; Protein: 2g; Total
Carbohydrates: 11g; Fiber: 7g; Fat: 14g

MACROS: 5% Protein; 72% Fat; 23% Carbohydrates

"Dress It Up" Salad Dressing

PREP TIME: 5 minutes • **MAKES 1 CUP**

Having a tasty salad dressing on hand will change how you think about salads. This easy spin on a classic vinaigrette is versatile and stores well. I also like to mix up the vinegar I add—I used balsamic vinegar for Weeknight Steak Salad (page 117) and light, tangy apple cider vinegar for Chickpea and Pear Kale Salad (page 84).

½ cup olive oil

½ cup balsamic or apple cider vinegar

2 teaspoons Dijon mustard

1 tablespoon honey (optional)

1 teaspoon salt

½ teaspoon freshly ground black pepper

1. Combine the olive oil, vinegar, Dijon, honey (if using), salt, and pepper in a jar with a tight-fitting lid.

2. Shake vigorously until well combined. Use immediately or refrigerate for up to 1 month.

FAT LOSS: If you're looking for more tang and less sweetness, you can easily omit the honey or lessen the amount you add, lowering the carbs.

PER SERVING (2 TABLESPOONS): Calories: 121; Protein: 0g; Total Carbohydrates: 2g; Fiber: 0g; Fat: 13g

---

MACROS: 0% Protein; 99% Fat; 1% Carbohydrates

Better-for-You Ranch Dip

PREP TIME: 5 minutes • **SERVES 4**

Making a healthful take on ranch can be fast and easy while still being extremely flavorful and packed with protein. Here, Greek yogurt replaces the mayonnaise or sour cream traditionally used in ranch dressing, the olive oil provides healthy unsaturated fats, and the herbs will remind you of the versions you grew up with. It's great as a dressing for salads and as a dip for veggies.

¾ cup plain low- or nonfat
  Greek yogurt

3 tablespoons olive oil

1 tablespoon minced fresh
  parsley

1 tablespoon minced fresh dill

1 tablespoon minced fresh
  chives

¼ teaspoon salt

1 tablespoon freshly squeezed
  lemon juice

1 garlic clove, minced

1. In a small bowl, combine the yogurt, olive oil, parsley, dill, chives, salt, lemon juice, and garlic. Whisk or stir to combine. You could also make this in a blender or food processor.

2. Serve immediately, or store in a sealed glass jar in the refrigerator for up to 1 month.

FAT LOSS: Greek yogurt is high in protein, so pairing it with veggies or using it as a dressing for salads is a great way to meet your macro targets.

PER SERVING (2 TABLESPOONS): Calories: 125; Protein: 2g; Total Carbohydrates: 4g; Fiber: 0g; Fat: 12g

MACROS: 6% Protein; 84% Fat; 10% Carbohydrates

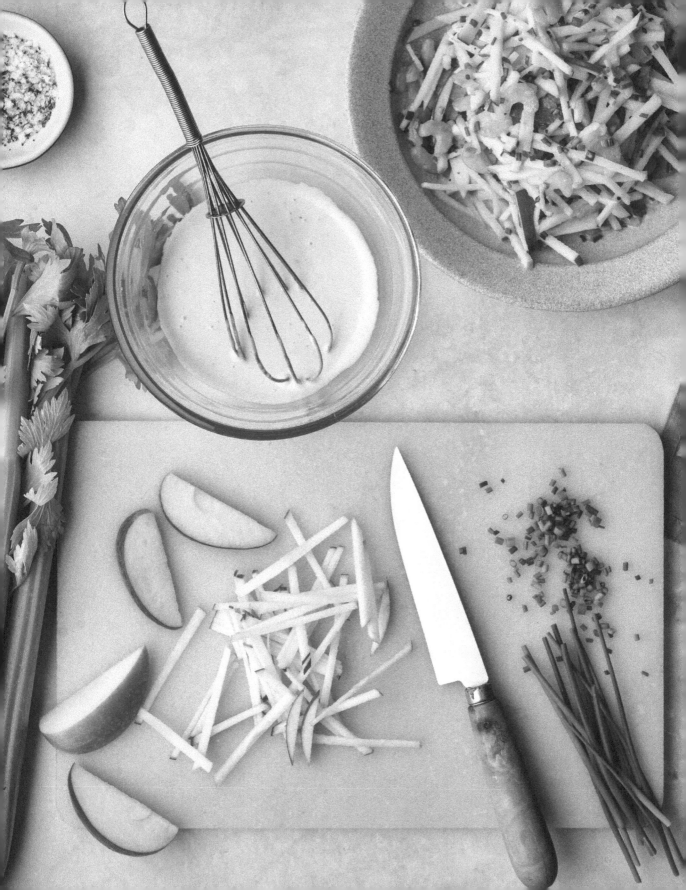

WORKOUT ROUTINES

Fat Loss

To support the goal of fat loss, there are two components I emphasize with my clients to help them succeed. The first and most important component is diet. In chapter 1, we reviewed in detail the importance of good food choices to support your health goals. The second component to promote fat loss is a combination of various exercises. Focusing on low-impact cardio, such as walking, rowing, or biking in addition to HIIT and strength training, is important to increase your metabolism while preventing muscle loss.

CARDIO

Work at a medium intensity at least 75 percent of the time. The goal is to keep you heart rate elevated, but not to the point of muscle failure or extreme fatigue.

- Walk on a flat or inclined surface for 30 minutes.

- Run or row for 20 to 30 minutes.

- Bike for 45 to 60 minutes.

    HIIT: *Do each of the following activities for 40 seconds on, followed by 20 seconds rest. Repeat 5 to 10 times. If you're just getting started, start with a goal of 5 rounds to complete your workout. Work up to 10 rounds as you advance in your physical activity.*

- Jumping Jacks

- Jump rope

- Burpees or Mountain Climbers

STRENGTH TRAINING

ROUTINE 1:

- Warm-up stretching

- Wall Sit – 1 minute (work up to 3 minutes) **1**

- 10 Burpees **2**

- Glute Bridge – 10 up and down, then hold for 30 seconds **3**

- 10 Push-Ups **4**

- Bicycle Crunches – 15 each leg **5**

- Cooldown stretching

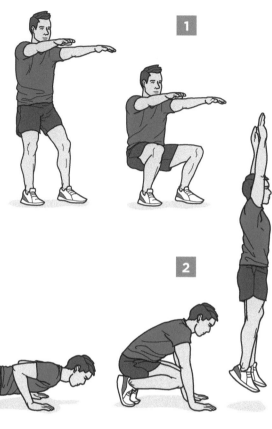

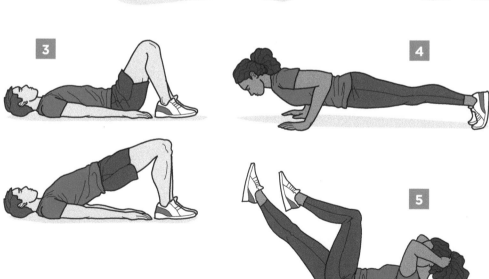

ROUTINE 2:

- Warm-up stretching
- 15 Squats **1**
- 20 Triceps Dips **2**
- Front Lunges – 10 each leg **3**
- 25 Jumping Jacks **4**
- Plank – 30 seconds (work up to 1 minute) **5**
- Cooldown stretching

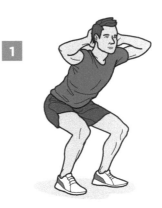

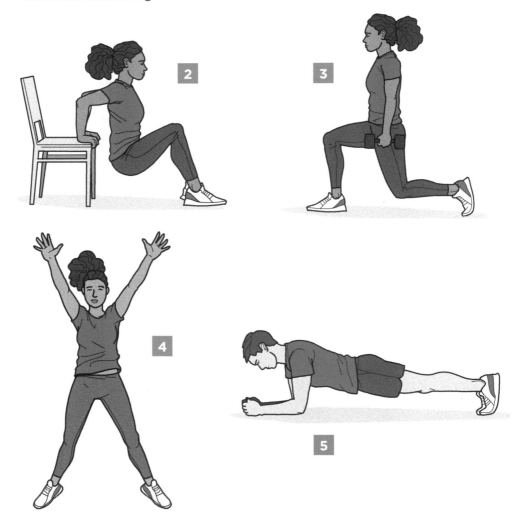

ROUTINE 3:

- Warm-up stretching
- 15 Squats **1**
- 15 Shoulder Presses **2**
- Mountain Climbers – 1 minute **3**
- 15 Bent-Over Rows **4**
- 10 Hollow Rocks **5**
- Cooldown stretching

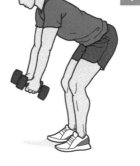

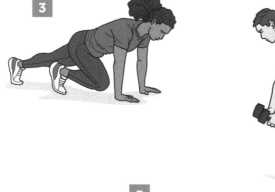

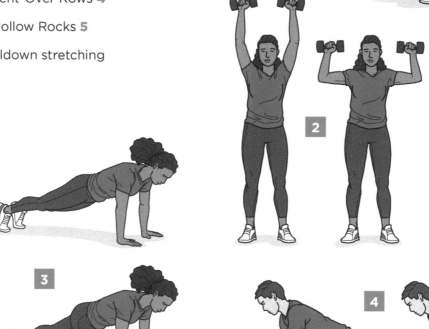

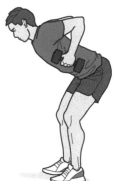

Muscle Gain

Support your muscle gain goals with a combination of strength training to build muscle mass and specific cardio exercises to help you burn fat. One of the most important takeaways with muscle gain goals is to ensure that you're feeding your body what it needs to recover and regenerate for each workout. When combining an intense strength training routine and cardio, your nutrition demands are high. Consuming enough protein and carbohydrates is critical to minimize the risk of plateaus and muscle fatigue.

CARDIO

When compared to fat loss, cardio exercises for muscle gain tend to be shorter but higher intensity. Aim to push yourself for 20 minutes, given the shorter duration.

- Walk at a fast pace for 20 minutes.

- Alternate medium jog or light run for 20 minutes.

- Row or stair-step for 20 minutes.

  HIIT: *To promote muscle building, I like the Every Minute on the Minute (EMOM) approach. Perform 10 of the following exercises for 45 seconds on with a 15-second rest, every minute on the minute, for 10 minutes.*

- Burpees

- Walking Lunges

- Sprints (sprint for 30 seconds, walk for 30 seconds). Do this for 10 minutes as a modified EMOM.

STRENGTH TRAINING

Start these strength training exercises with just your body weight. As you get more comfortable with the exercises, you can begin to add hand weights. Be sure that your form is solid before adding weight, as moving too quickly can result in injury.

ROUTINE 1:

- Warm-up stretching
- 15 Squats **1**
- 20 Triceps Dips **2**
- Front Lunges – 10 each leg **3**
- 25 Jumping Jacks **4**
- Plank – 30 seconds (work up to 1 minute) **5**
- Cooldown stretching

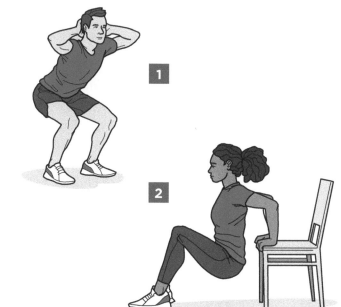

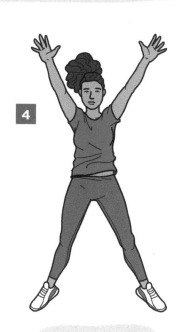

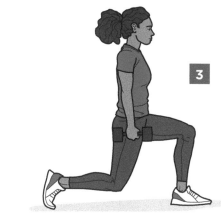

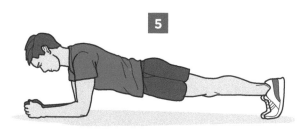

ROUTINE 2:

- Warm-up stretching
- Wall Sit – 1 minute (work up to 3 minutes) **1**
- 10 Burpees **2**
- Glute Bridge – 10 up and down, then hold for 30 seconds **3**
- 10 Push-Ups **4**
- Bicycle Crunches – 15 each leg **5**
- Cooldown stretching

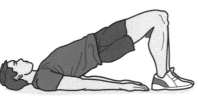

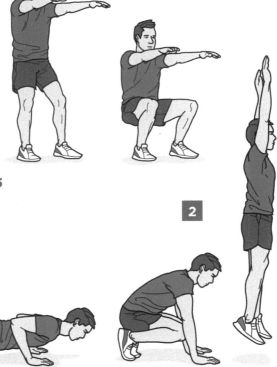

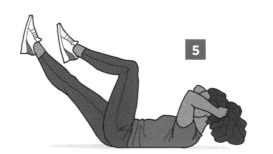

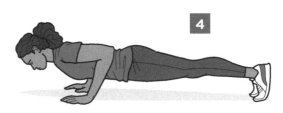

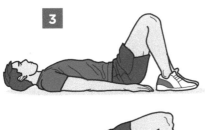

ROUTINE 3:

- Warm-up stretching
- 15 Squats **1**
- 15 Shoulder Presses **2**
- Mountain Climbers – 1 minute **3**
- 15 Bent-Over Rows **4**
- 10 Hollow Rocks **5**
- Cooldown stretching

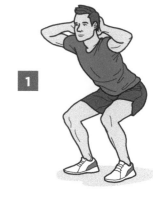

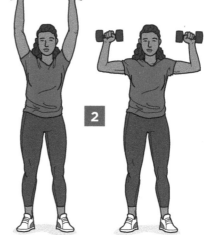

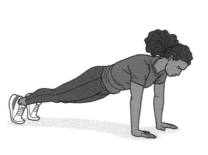

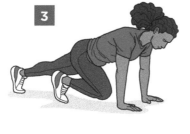

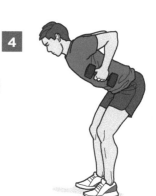

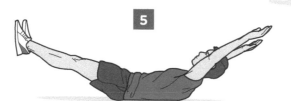

MEASUREMENT CONVERSIONS

VOLUME EQUIVALENTS (LIQUID)

US STANDARD	US STANDARD (OUNCES)	METRIC (APPROX.)
2 tablespoons	1 fl. oz.	30 mL
¼ cup	2 fl. oz.	60 mL
½ cup	4 fl. oz.	120 mL
1 cup	8 fl. oz.	240 mL
1½ cups	12 fl. oz.	355 mL
2 cups or 1 pint	16 fl. oz.	475 mL
4 cups or 1 quart	32 fl. oz.	1 L
1 gallon	128 fl. oz.	4 L

OVEN TEMPERATURES

FAHRENHEIT (F)	CELSIUS (C) (APPROX.)
250°	120°
300°	150°
325°	165°
350°	180°
375°	190°
400°	200°
425°	220°
450°	230°

VOLUME EQUIVALENTS (DRY)

US STANDARD	METRIC (APPROX.)
⅛ teaspoon	0.5 mL
¼ teaspoon	1 mL
½ teaspoon	2 mL
¾ teaspoon	4 mL
1 teaspoon	5 mL
1 tablespoon	15 mL
¼ cup	59 mL
⅓ cup	79 mL
½ cup	118 mL
⅔ cup	156 mL
¾ cup	177 mL
1 cup	235 mL
2 cups or 1 pint	475 mL
3 cups	700 mL
4 cups or 1 quart	1 L

WEIGHT EQUIVALENTS

US STANDARD	METRIC (APPROX.)
½ ounce	15 g
1 ounce	30 g
2 ounces	60 g
4 ounces	115 g
8 ounces	225 g
12 ounces	340 g
16 ounces or 1 pound	455 g

REFERENCES

Centers for Disease Control and Prevention. "Micronutrient Facts." Last modified February 2022. cdc.gov/nutrition/micronutrient-malnutrition/micronutrients.

Halton, Thomas L., and Frank B. Hu. "The Effects of High Protein Diets on Thermogenesis, Satiety, and Weight Loss: A Critical Review." *Journal of the American College of Nutrition* 23, no. 5 (2004): 373–85. doi:10.108%7315724.2004.10719381.

International Atomic Energy Agency. "Diet Quality." iaea.org/topics/diet-quality.

Krzysztofik, Michal, Michal Wilk, Grzegorz Wojdała, and Artur Gołaś. "Maximizing Muscle Hypertrophy: A Systematic Review of Advanced Resistance Training Techniques and Methods" *International Journal of Environmental Research and Public Health* 16, no. 24 (2019): 4897. doi:10.3390/ijerph16244897.

Mifflin, M. D., et al. "A New Predictive Equation for Resting Energy Expenditure in Healthy Individuals." *American Journal of Clinical Nutrition* 51, no. 2 (1990): 241–7. doi:10.1093/ajcn/51.2.241.

National Institutes of Health, Office of Dietary Supplements. "Calcium Fact Sheet for Consumers." Last modified November 17, 2021. ods.od.nih.gov/factsheets/Calcium-Consumer.

National Institutes of Health, Office of Dietary Supplements. "Iron Fact Sheet for Consumers." Last modified March 22, 2021. ods.od.nih.gov/factsheets/Iron-Consumer.

National Institutes of Health, Office of Dietary Supplements. "Vitamin A Fact Sheet for Consumers." Last modified January 14, 2021. ods.od.nih.gov /factsheets/VitaminA-Consumer.

National Institutes of Health, Office of Dietary Supplements. "Vitamin D Fact Sheet for Consumers." Last modified March 22, 2021. ods.od.nih.gov /factsheets/VitaminD-Consumer.

National Institutes of Health, Office of Dietary Supplements. "Zinc Fact Sheet for Consumers." Last modified December 8, 2021. ods.od.nih.gov /factsheets/Zinc-Consumer.

National Research Council (US) Committee on Diet and Health. *Diet and Health: Implications for Reducing Chronic Disease Risk.* Washington (DC): National Academies Press (US); 1989.

Wolfe, Robert R., et al. "Optimizing Protein Intake in Adults: Interpretation and Application of the Recommended Dietary Allowance Compared with the Acceptable Macronutrient Distribution Range." *Advances in Nutrition (Bethesda, Md.)* 8, no. 2 (2017): 266–275. doi:10.3945/an.116.013821.

INDEX

Acknowledgments

I would first and foremost like to thank my husband for his support during the book writing process. Eric, this book would not have been completed without your questions, listening ear, recipe ideas, and willingness to taste-test. For that, thank you. I would also like to thank my editor, Marjorie DeWitt, who guided me in this entire process, answering all my questions and supporting me throughout; and Callisto, for believing in me and providing me with the wonderful opportunity to share my knowledge and expertise with readers everywhere.

About the Author

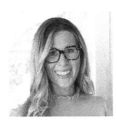 **BRITTANY SCANNIELLO, RDN,** is an award-winning registered dietitian. She received her undergraduate degree in Human Nutrition and Dietetics from University of North Carolina at Greensboro and completed her dietetic internship at UC Davis Medical Center in California. Scanniello has worked in both hospital and industry settings in clinical nutrition and, most recently, in her own Colorado-based integrative nutrition company and private practice, Eat Simply Nutrition. As a lifelong and collegiate athlete, she focuses on sports and functional nutrition.

Scanniello is a respected voice in the community and has contributed to a number of publications as a freelance writer, guest blogger, and nutrition expert. She resides in Lafayette, Colorado, with her two daughters, her husband, and their poodle, Leonard.

CPSIA information can be obtained
at www.ICGtesting.com
Printed in the USA
JSHW060717161122
33229JS00001B/1